THE 90 DAY CIO

STRATEGIES FOR OPTIMIZING OUTCOMES AND VALUE

Dr. Luis E. Taveras, PhD

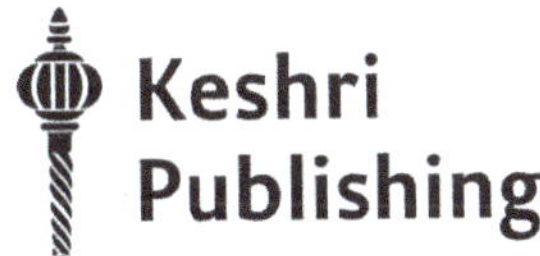

Keshri
Publishing

Dedicated to Beth, my wife of four decades, and our children, Christopher, Alicia, and Danny. Your unwavering support regardless of what I've decided to do has been the cornerstone of my success.
Thank you for your encouragement, patience and most of all, your love!

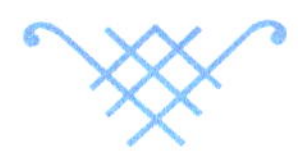

The 90 Day CIO Model© by Dr. Luis E. Taveras, PhD

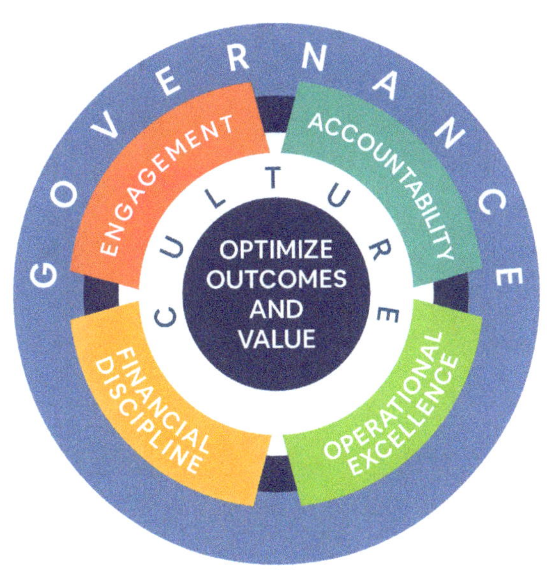

Table of Contents

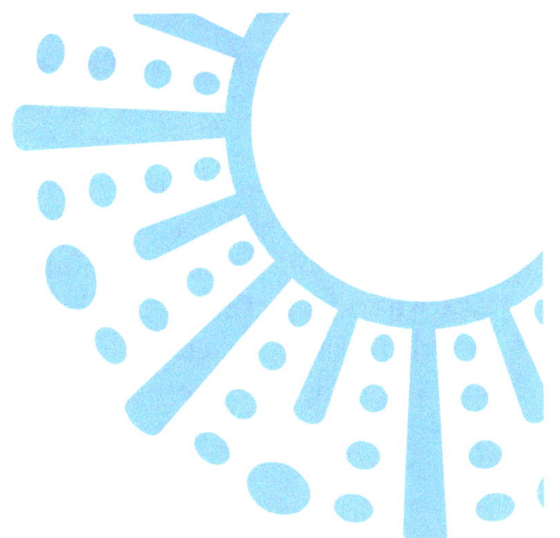

PREFACE:

Leading Change (Personal and Professional) as an Executive

On September 11th, 2001, at 9:03am, I stood on the corner of 12th Street and 6th Avenue and watched a passenger plane smash into the South Tower of the World Trade Center…

A few minutes earlier I was sitting with one of my project managers at St. Vincent's hospital. The first hijacked plane flew by, and I said something glib, like, "this guy must be lost." We always had air traffic near the hospital, so we were used to seeing and hearing planes go by, but this one felt unusually close.

Then the phone call came through to advise me that there was a "mass emergency" and that we were to prepare for significant casualties arriving imminently.

I put two and two together and I left the hospital to see what had happened. Sure enough, I could see the plane lodged in the corner of one of the Twin Towers and thick, black smoke filling the sky. When the second plane came into view, it never even occurred to me what was going to happen next. My imagination couldn't conjure up this level of horror. I remember thinking, "Oh, this plane must be going to see what's happened to the first one." It was an odd thought, but it had barely registered when the South Tower was struck, and I heard the kind of almighty explosion that only occurs when two solid structures briefly attempt to occupy the same space.

St. Vincent's has a long, famous history of dealing with historic tragedies. When it was founded in the 19th century it coincided with the cholera epidemic that killed between 5-10% of people in large cities, including New York which was the first US city to be significantly affected. In 1912, survivors of the Titanic were shipped to St. Vincent's for treatment. And in the 1980s, St. Vincent's established the first AIDS ward on the East Coast.

As the closest level-one trauma center to the World Trade Center, 9/11 became the latest in a long line of monumental moments in the history of the hospital. And I was thrust into the middle of it.

At the time I was the Senior Vice President and Chief Technology Officer of Saint Vincent's Catholic Medical Centers. Part of my role was to lead in a time of crisis and this definitely qualified. I raced back to the hospital to make preparations, and although I didn't typically participate in an active mass emergency, the scale of this event meant that virtually every member of the hospital's staff, regardless of their role or medical training, was pulled in to help out.

We had actually practiced mass casualty situations before, but this was on a scale that was unprecedented. For example, I quickly realized that we were unlikely to have enough stretchers to manage the volume of patients that were likely already heading our way. I started sending people into offices to grab anything they could find with wheels – office chairs and the like. That was as much as I managed before the first of the injured began to arrive.

The initial wave of patients were the people hit by falling jet fuel that landed around the towers. The burns were horrific, and we had to treat them quickly. After that, people were arriving by any means possible. Walking, taxis, private vehicles, police cars. As the closest trauma center, almost everyone who survived the initial impacts and were physically able to leave the area were being brought to us.

Of course, it was chaos, but I'm proud of the way in which everyone pulled together and improvised. For instance, it was a simple thing, but because there was only one main entrance to the ER, and we had people arriving in hurry, and at the same time people leaving to try to help out on the street, it was creating a bottleneck. So, I made the call to open up the garage and direct people to use this as an exit. The main entrance became purely for people entering, and the garage for people leaving. That helped to keep the flow of people moving and allowed us to get patients to the treatment areas faster.

I am a planner. I like plans. I like back-up plans. I like my back-up plans to have back-up plans. But I don't know how you could ever plan for something like this. I feel privileged to have been in a position to help on that day, but at the same time it's a terrible memory to live with.

When the events first began unfolding, I had the presence of mind to call my wife and let her know that I was okay. But after that it was impossible for her to get hold of me for a long time. And then she began hearing stories of people who had called home to say that they were okay but had suddenly gone missing because the call was in between the two tower strikes, or because they'd survived the plane crashes, but were killed by falling debris when the buildings collapsed.

My wife took the kids out of school, and they had an anxious wait, watching things unfold on the news. Incredibly, they were able to confirm that I was okay because, by chance, they saw me on a news report, right outside the front of the ER, a nebulizer in my hand. Still, the waiting and the worrying, trying to make sense of the senseless violence that had taken place. No one can go through that experience, whether directly because you were there, or indirectly because friends of family or work colleagues were there, and not be scarred.

Despite the chaos, most of the patients coming to the ER had relatively minor physical injuries. Which meant the ER was never really overwhelmed. Sadly, most of the people in the vicinity of the attack either walked away with fairly light injuries... or they died.

Perhaps that's the best way to illustrate just how dark this day was, not just for the US, but for the whole world.

If I had to live that day over, knowing what I know now, would I have done things differently? Probably. But to be honest I don't care to think about it from that perspective.

What I prefer is to look back on that day and consider two things. What did I learn from that experience? And what was it about my abilities and prior experience that equipped me to deal with this? I am telling you this because, when I answer those questions, I get right down to the root of what this book is really about.

It is Not About The Tech

Yes, this book is about the modern face of the Chief Information Officer (CIO) role in the world of healthcare. But ironically, technology is not the true foundation of this role, this book, or the 90-Day CIO strategy.

Ultimately, the beating heart of the modern CIO is people and the care that we provide them. Whether it's a 75-year-old lady on palliative care who wants to live out her remaining days at home. A 12-year-old child with leukemia who has a phobia of needles. A nurse in a beyond-capacity care home, anxious about not having enough time to spend with each resident. A chief surgeon who wants to perform pioneering surgery but is struggling to make a business case to purchase the equipment she needs. In every case, there is a unique person who deserves to be treated with care and understanding.

Technology can serve these people well, but it is merely a means to an end.

On 9/11, when news traveled about a horrific incident at the World Trade Center, volunteers began arriving from all over the city. Medical students and physicians on vacation in New York were showing up ready to roll up their sleeves and help wherever they could.

It was heart-warming and it was valuable, but it also created a new logistical challenge. Because now a hospital already flooded with people was becoming dangerously overcrowded. It would have been easy to just start turning volunteers away, but to do so would have been to forget that these were also grieving, distraught people who were desperate to be useful. I ended up directing all volunteers to the cafeteria and we set up a system there to manage people as they arrived and figure out in what ways they could help.

When you work in healthcare you cannot, under any circumstances, afford to lose sight of the fact that the end goal is the health and wellbeing of the people involved, whether it be the people being treated or the people providing the treatment. Even when things get hectic and you're in a senior position that requires you to take more of a birds-eye, almost abstract, view of what's unfolding, you must never forget that ultimately, it's the people that matter.

That perspective was critical to my ability to be effective on that fateful day. Every time I was called on to make a decision and find an approach to a problem, I made myself take a breath and think about what was best for the people around me.

So, in the afternoon, when people began showing up with pictures of missing loved ones and asking for help to find them, I instructed the staff not to dismiss them, not to tell them that we were too busy, and absolutely under no circumstances to make them feel the situation was hopeless. Instead, they were to take the picture, thank them, and promise we would do everything we could.

When people are desperate and panicking, more than anything else they need to feel that they are doing something useful and productive, no matter how small or potentially fruitless it may prove to be. Taking a photograph from a terrified person who is desperately looking for a loved one and thanking them was a small offering, but it was a way to treat that person with kindness and dignity.

I can think of no circumstances when that isn't the right approach to take.

When an unforeseen crisis threatens to overwhelm you and the healthcare system you work for, organization is critical, seeing the big picture is important, and thinking ahead is key...

...but none of that can replace or outweigh putting the needs of the people first.

If you've been a CIO for any length of time, you likely already know this to be true. Your focus may be on the technology, but only because it's a means to an end. The goal isn't to have the best tech because we like shiny new objects, but because, if the right tool is selected for the right job, the end result is the ability to improve health and save lives.

My conclusion is that it's these determined beliefs that enabled me to operate well on what will likely be the most stressful and catastrophic situation in which I will ever find myself. And it served to confirm my belief that the people, and the care you provide them, is what will get you to where you need to be in your career as a CIO.

The CIO is Dead... Long Live The CIO

My motivation for writing this book is to address, head on, the reality that the traditional application of the CIO role has gone. It is dead. Or at the very least redundant. That is not to say that a CIO cannot still cling desperately to the old ways of doing things, but if you do so your career is probably living on borrowed time.

The old methods of handling a CIO role, especially in healthcare, are totally inadequate to serve an industry and a world scene that is changing at a pace never before seen in history. All aspects of the healthcare industry are going through major transformations, and if you try to tackle new challenges with old methods, you're going to find yourself increasingly moving away from putting the health of patients at the forefront of the minds and goals of every person in your department.

This book will address every area of the CIO role that needs to be adjusted and updated to reflect this new paradigm, but the most significant element that threads its way into every part of the 90-Day CIO strategy is this:

You need to go from being reactive… to being proactive.

Heaven forbid you ever have to experience anything on the scale of 9/11 for yourself, but the only way to be confident that you can handle anything the healthcare industry can throw at you is to have a system and an infrastructure that is designed to quickly adapt and flex to a change in circumstances without falling apart.

It's not about imagining every worst-case scenario and making a contingency plan. That will only get you so far. At St. Vincent's we prepared and practiced for crises, but nothing could fully prepare us for the chaos on the streets outside our hospital on 9/11. Nothing. I believe I handled that situation only because my personality type, my education and my career choices had taught me how to adjust quickly and plot a course through the confusion.

The 90-Day CIO strategy is going to give you a version of this resilience and this forward-thinking that will allow you to develop a high-performing healthcare network. Not because you have an unassailable ability to predict the future, but because you've created excellence across every team and every department for which you're responsible.

And if 90 days sounds like too short a time to accomplish this… you are absolutely right. In reality this is more likely to be a journey that takes closer to five years. Maybe a little less, maybe a little more – depending on the size of your operation and the shape it's currently in – but everything is going to grow out of those first 90 days.

The truth is, there is no single set of healthcare CIO operations I can give you that will work everywhere, all of the time. The end result is going to vary depending on your location, the resources you have available, your budget, the size of the organization you're running, and the breadth of your oversight. I can't give you a one-size-fits-all.

What I will give you, however, is a 90-day journey that will allow you to set the foundation for everything that comes next. You'll put systems in place that will start to change the way in which progress happens. You'll develop communication practices that eliminate black holes of understanding among your staff. You'll create new mind-sets among your team members that will support your vision and ensure buy-in from everyone involved in this project.

Within 90 days you'll have a crystal-clear view of where you are, where you need to be, and what it's going to take to get you there.

A Word of Warning...

Before you turn the page and begin your 90-day journey into CIO excellence, take a breath and ask yourself whether you are ready to initiate change across virtually every area of your authority.

You know without me even telling you that this journey is going to require some substantial changes, not just for you but for the people that work alongside you and under you. Maybe that makes you nervous, or maybe you're just fine with it. But either way, you need to interrogate your attitude toward change because how YOU deal with it is going to have a sizable impact on how everyone else deals with it.

Simply put, if you're not comfortable with the changes you decide to make, even to a small degree, the people around you will pick up on this and you're going to witness anxiety, resistance, and even anger.

The journey of a modern CIO in healthcare typically requires change in virtually every department and process, so unsurprisingly this book contains an entire chapter on how to manage change effectively and how to gain the support of everyone else who will be impacted by this journey. But what this book can't do is give you the right mindset that is needed to kick off this program. That part is down to you.

It is not enough to shrug and think, 'I'm not a fan of change; but I'm tough, I'll manage, I'll get through it…" That isn't going to get the job done. Any internal resistance or anxiety around change is going to be magnified in the people around you ten-fold.

So, start thinking about this now. Think deeply about how you feel about the unknown and about breaking new ground. If it helps, talk to a respected colleague or a loved one and ask them how they feel you deal with change. And once you are mentally prepared to tackle this journey without hesitation or equivocation, then and only then should you embark on your 90-day journey.

I'm confident you're up for the challenge. You wouldn't be reading this book if you weren't the kind of forward-thinking, bold individual who recognizes the value of personal and business development and is willing to take on a tough project that is going to ultimately allow you to better serve your patients and your staff.

If there's any benefit to personally going through the kind of horrific event that I experienced on 9/11, it's that surviving such an event adds a layer of steel to your psyche that can't really be obtained in any other way. I would never wish for you to go through anything like that level of trauma, but what I can do is gift to you the lessons I've gained through this experience and many other challenging moments in my career in healthcare.

My comfort with change and my ability to rise above the chaos, and embrace it, has allowed me to thrive through over forty years in IT and healthcare. I am uniquely equipped to instruct and inspire you on this journey and I'm grateful for the opportunity to do so.

Taming chaos and gaining control of even the most difficult moments is the daily challenge of the modern CIO in healthcare. And if you don't do it, nobody else will.

Go ahead and do whatever mental preparations you feel you need to do to get your head in the game and embark on what is going to be the most exciting and fulfilling period in your career.

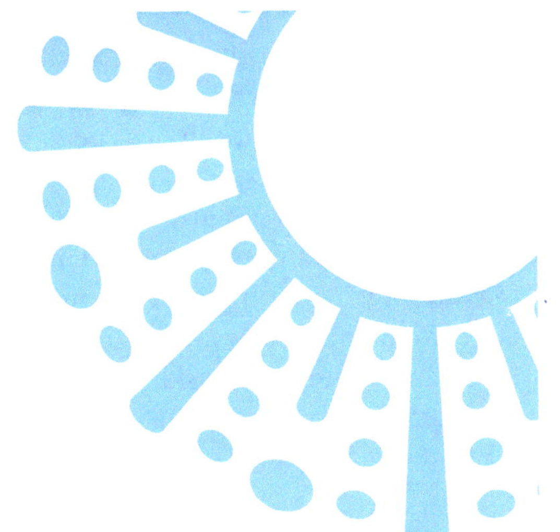

CHAPTER ONE

The Evolution of the CIO to Change Agent

At some point during the last couple of decades we all just quietly accepted that we're living in a sci-fi novel. Tablets, smartwatches, voice-enabled assistants, 3D-printing, cloud computing, artificial intelligence – these are all technologies that weren't supposed to arrive until the starship Enterprise began boldly going where no one had gone before. And yet, not only do these technologies exist at a consumer-level, but they're also so commonplace we no longer even marvel at them.

Technology in healthcare is no different. Exoskeletons, neurostimulation, 3D-printed drugs, genome editing, medical wearables, robotic surgery – again all innovations that were envisioned when I was younger, but that seem to have arrived at far greater speed than most would have predicted.

When I first started working in healthcare, we would input records into massive mainframe computers with green and black monitors and print out the results onto green and white, continuous form paper. Now we use wireless touchscreen devices, connected to cloud storage that can hold petabytes of information with ease.

But it's not just the technology that has rapidly advanced; the systems around them have had to adapt alongside it. If you have any gray hair, you probably remember the days when resolving a computer problem meant grabbing Dave from IT as you passed him in the cafeteria and asking him to take a look. No record-keeping, no systemization, no best practices – just a few guys troubleshooting as and when required.

It is this massive leap forward in technology that has made the CIO role in healthcare both exciting and extremely challenging. Because it's not just the complexity of the tech that we have to deal with, but also the accompanying shift in how the tech is used, the departments that use it (long gone are the days when it was purely used by administrators), the expectations from staff and patients, as well as the potential for great financial and productivity gains. And, of course, the potential for great harm if misused.

This has not been a gradual evolution through the steady gains of natural selection, but more akin to punctuated equilibrium. It would be as if yesterday we just learned to cross the oceans, and tomorrow we make plans to fly to Mars.

If you think I'm exaggerating, even a little, you haven't been paying attention. Artificial intelligence and machine learning are going to power a revolution in predictive healthcare, brain mapping is going to transform our ability to treat disorders such as autism and Alzheimer's, and surgically implanted stimulators are going to return mobility to people with spinal cord injuries. Technology advancement in healthcare hasn't peaked or plateaued, it's barely begun. In fact, I've probably made a big mistake in naming the above predicted advances because likely, even in just a few years, what I've just said may sound quaint.

But now the awkward question that I need you to ask yourself, and to do so with complete candor…

Don't be alarmed if you find the answer is the latter. It would be almost impossible for the answer to be anything else. But as I highlighted in the previous chapter, if there have been no significant changes, you're a long way from acting with any worthwhile efficiency. Think of the above question as a way to highlight why so many CIOs in healthcare struggle to keep pace, remain organized, or make effective use of their budget.

It's only once you fully appreciate the root cause of a problem that you can really begin to repair it. And in this instance, the root cause is using analogue systems in a digital world.

So, try to relax. Even if you have been in this line of work for many years, you're a long way from being obsolete. Really, if anyone is out of date, it should be me. After four decades in the industry – at least half of that in CIO roles – I should be the crustiest of dinosaurs. The fact that I'm not obsolete should be an indicator that age has nothing to do with it.

I am actually the opposite. I've stayed on the cutting-edge of healthcare technology and the modern strategies needed to manage any paradigm throughout my career. I've been driving changes through

CIO roles that have allowed my employers to keep pace with the advances in tech, as well as dramatic changes in the health and social make-up of our society. For example:

- ✦ At Saint Vincent's I managed the CTO role in a $1.5B operation taking in 8 hospitals, as well as numerous nursing homes, primary care clinics and behavioral health facilities.

- ✦ At Accenture I played a key leadership role in winning outsourcing opportunities exceeding $500M in contract value.

- ✦ At Barnabas Health I handled the CIO role while also juggling the Senior Vice President position, leading two Accountable Care Organizations, and driving the implementation of a systemwide influenza immunization program among other significant operations.

- ✦ And most recently, I cared for the CIO role for the entire City of Buffalo, the second largest city in the state of New York, with a population of 260,000 people.

I share these roles with you, not to brag, but to illustrate that the systems and practices I'm going to be sharing in this book are proven to produce excellence in roles of the largest size and complexity. There's no need to be daunted by the scope of the challenge you're facing. The 90-Day CIO strategy is designed to flex to whatever shape and mass your organization might take.

While other healthcare networks struggle to keep up with the pace of change and continue to find black holes between the capabilities of the tech they own and how they're actually being used, by the end of this process you'll be ahead of the curve and have a comfortable grasp of everything within your purview. But that is not all…

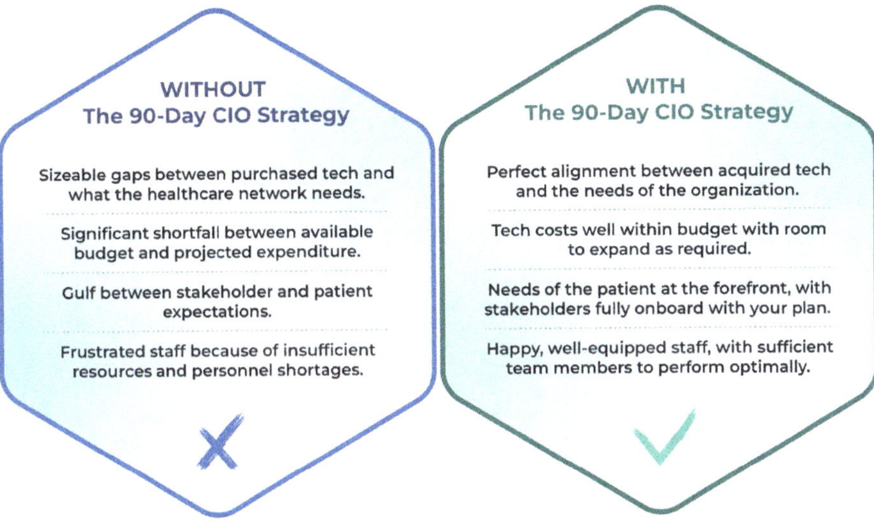

Figure 1.1 A comparison of outcomes with and without the 90 Day CIO Strategy.

I don't want to sidetrack too much by digging into the above results now – we'll cover all of these in more detail along the way – but I want to briefly highlight the second item in the second box, which touches on the challenges of matching your assigned budget with what you need to achieve your targets. This area is huge because it affects, not just the tech you're able to purchase, but your ability to keep sufficient resources to manage your position and keep your team motivated.

Now, more than ever, it seems that whenever a large organization has to engage in cost-cutting exercises, the speed with which it progresses to laying off staff has accelerated. I'm not saying that this is never an unfortunate but necessary step, but I do believe that often more can and should be done to avoid this step. We can't put people at the heart of our role as CIO and not do everything in our power to avoid putting people out of a job. This is not about sentimentality; it's about dignifying the people that we work with. But equally, it's about acknowledging the simple fact that reducing employee numbers often does more harm to morale among those remaining, while simultaneously causing great harm to the organization's ability to serve its patients.

This is just one of the things that is going to change when you've completed the 90-Day CIO strategy. You'll have the mindset to resist pressure to lay-off staff, and the strategies to find other ways to tackle budget deficits.

Time and time again, I've been successful in creating forward-thinking, high-performance IT programs in massive healthcare networks that are robust, well-designed, and measurably adding value to patient healthcare outcomes. And that is what you are also going to accomplish if you follow this process.

The Modern CIO (AKA - the Change Agent)

There are few things more tempting than holding a well-paid senior role, sliding into a comfortable rut, and making sure everything is just about good enough (as long as no one looks too closely). But I have never fallen into that trap. Quite the opposite. I've managed to stay at the forefront of healthcare technology and the significant demands of the CIO role, and never allowed myself to get too comfortable and start resisting change.

How? Maybe it's just how I was built.

I was born in the Dominican Republic, but I came to the United States in 1970. I was 12 years old, and it was my first time in an airplane, so the whole thing was really exciting. But it was also a very big change. I flew into JFK in March, so the weather was perfectly fine, but for me it felt noticeably cool compared to what I was used to.

And we were a big family. It took time to get everything sorted out. For a while there were ten of us living in a one-bedroom apartment in the South Bronx. Imagine that! Then, of course, I had to get accustomed to going to school where the culture and language and environment was very different. But even through that challenge of being a fish out of Caribbean waters, my abilities as a student were noticed. I was introduced to the program, A Better Chance (ABC), which helps place high-performing minority students from inner cities in high-profile schools.

I was offered a placement at New Canaan High School in New Canaan, Connecticut which was a fabulous opportunity, but it was a big decision. It would have been easy to say, "Oh, this isn't for me. I can't be away from my mom and my sisters. I'm still getting used to living in a new country. I'm Hispanic, I'm going to feel out of place. Heck, I'm still getting used to eating American food."

It would have been easy to say those things, but I didn't. I may have thought some of them, but in the end, I knew a great opportunity when I saw it. These kinds of chances don't come along very often – sometimes never – especially for a young immigrant in a low-income family. It would never have seriously occurred to me not to seize this life-changing offer that was being handed to me.

Was it easy? No, of course not. When I went home for that first Thanksgiving holiday, it took a serious effort to make myself go back because it was hard leaving my family behind again. But in time I adjusted and there's no question that the ABC program helped me take my first steps toward the successful career that followed. At the time of writing, I'm soon going to be heading back to New Canaan for my 45th high school reunion where I graduated in the top ten percent of my class and was inducted into the National Honor Society.

You can see where I'm going with this story, right? It is a story about change. A change in country, a change in language, a change in housing, a change in culture, a change in schooling. But I didn't focus on the change, I focused on the opportunities. Sometimes people are given the chance to do something new and amazing with their life, but they don't take it – in fact they may not even register it as an opportunity – because all they're seeing is that this is going to involve change, which is potentially going to be difficult and unsettling. But if you learn to see past the change and see the amazing things that can come out at the other end, you start to see change, not as a burden, but as a window of exciting possibilities.

This mindset that I was unintentionally developing first found its fruition at International Business Machines (IBM). While I was in college, I was pre-med and very busy with my studies, but like many students I was open to working during the holidays to make some extra cash. The ABC program assigns its students a host family, and the husband in that family, a general manager at IBM, threw me some work over the summer. I didn't know it at the time, but this was going to be instrumental in my subsequent career choices.

Around about that time, IBM launched a new data entry machine, the 5280. This was before the mainstream adoption of the personal computer, so it still required programming knowledge to operate, but it was smaller, faster and more affordable than other similar machines on the market. There and then I decided I was going to become an expert in this device.

My logic was simple. The companies that needed this computer were, by definition, forward-thinking but very busy, and likely didn't have the time to learn all the ins and outs. If I became known as one of the few, or maybe only, true experts in this device, then I would *have* to be the one they called when they needed help. I'm not sure quite how fully-formed this concept was in my head, but I was already positioning myself as an expert consultant.

It was this work that steered me towards working in the tech industry, all the while maintaining my interest in health care. In my senior college year, I worked as a consultant for an American bank in New York on the weekend, pulling in $75 an hour (a huge sum for a college student in the late 70s). Once I graduated, I went to work for IBM, and by the late 80s I was the marketing manager for all healthcare in New Jersey. From there it was a few short steps to moving into my first CTO role at St. Vincent's Catholic Medical Centers in New York City.

It's not hard to draw a straight line from my combined interest and experience with tech and healthcare during my college years, to my two-decades long career in CIO roles. But what underpinned my progression, and my success was that eye for spotting opportunities, my understanding of the value of becoming an expert in something most people can't (or won't), and my appreciation that making the best use of tech and embracing change go hand in hand.

Was all of this planned out? Was it good fortune? Was it educated foresight? Whatever the reason, it left me perfectly placed to appreciate what a modern CIO needs to be able to do to excel, and to create a framework that allows them to succeed even under the most challenging of circumstances.

Like it or not, if you are going to become a truly progressive CIO in healthcare, you need to think of yourself, first and foremost, as a change agent. If you can't embrace change with rampant enthusiasm and generate similar levels of enthusiasm for change among the people you work alongside and the people you manage, you cannot be effective in your role. Worse, you could even begin to be a drain on the organization.

Technology has not finished changing. There's no eye of the storm in our future. So, you either roll with it, or you let the winds of change blow you away.

Being persuasive is one key part of being a change agent. Here are the others...

A true board member: Some c-level executives may view the CTO or CIO roles as being lesser. As if you're just a tech-head, sitting on the sidelines, waiting for the real managers to give you a project. Obviously, this isn't true, but you may unintentionally be giving that impression. After the next 90 days, no one will ever dare even think such a thing. You're going to be a proactive, vocal member of the board.

Involved in the full tech life cycle: In the past, you were primarily responsible for purchasing and maintaining computers, chiefly for the administration departments. But now that tech pervades every healthcare department, your oversight has increased to include identifying the needs of your organization, selecting the appropriate equipment, training the users, integrating the new devices with existing tech, and optimizing the output and success of your purchases.

Recognizing yourself as a unique leader: The healthcare CIO stands apart from most other CIO roles. There are few, if any, other industries that require the oversight of so many different forms of tech, including data processing for administration, medical equipment for doctors and surgeons, and wearables for patients. And the added wrinkle that the health and wellbeing of your patients is more important than turning a profit. Or if it isn't right now, it will be by the end of this process.

Comfortable with change: I won't rehash this because we've already discussed it at length. Suffices to say that "change" in this role includes changes in tech, healthcare needs, social pressures, and political environments.

A driver of change: It's not enough to be comfortable and enthusiastic about change. You must also inspire that attitude in those around you, especially among those members of your team, and even more among your fellow leadership team members. It's your job to figure out the short-term, medium-term, and long-term needs of your organization, and then convince your fellow managers because they need to agree with your conclusions.

The Pareto Imperative

One final word on the importance of embracing change as a modern healthcare CIO. Because although change is going to ripple through every move that you make in the next 90 days, I can think of no greater way of really driving home this point than highlighting what is going to become one of your chief goals over the next few months…

Moving the split in resources between supporting existing tech and its users and innovating the use of tech within your organization.

In the unlikely event that you're unfamiliar with it, the Pareto principle is the idea that around 80% of consequences tend to come from around 20% of the causes. Vilfredo Pareto developed the idea in the 19th century that 80% of the land in Italy was owned by 20% of the population. More recently the concept has been observed in a wide range of disparate fields, including sales, marketing, investing, sports, traffic, and even crime.

In this instance we can use it to describe the above split to say that in most industries, including healthcare, about 80% of the IT department's time and money goes into supporting and maintaining existing tech, while the other 20% goes into innovating and improving the tech.

This is totally unacceptable for a modern healthcare CIO. So, we're going to flip this on its head.

By the end of this journey (that's the next few years, not the next 90 days), you're going to be putting 20% of your resources into maintaining your tech and its users, and the other 80% into innovating and developing your tech.

If your knee jerk reaction is that this sounds totally unrealistic, you now know why I said this is the poster child for the level of change you're going to be masterminding.

There was a time when I used to promote a 50/50 split between the two, which even then used to generate some strong reactions. But to truly stay at the forefront of tech implementation and to keep your healthcare organization running at peak efficiency, you're going to need to be at 80/20.

Again, it bears repeating, this isn't going to happen overnight. You're going to need to change the way in which you oversee your departments, and you're going to need to change the habits of your team and the people that work for you. But you may also find it reassuring to consider that innovating and developing tech doesn't necessarily mean spending lots of money on new, shiny objects. The biggest part of this process is evolving what you already have so it is more efficient, coordinates better with other systems, experiences less downtime, and produces measurably better results for the users, and the end beneficiaries - i.e., the patients.

It's about moving your organization forward so it can achieve better results, which simply isn't possible if you're spending the vast majority of your time working feverishly just to keep things from breaking. Imagine a Formula One car construction team that spent 80% of their time keeping the car running and only 20% of their time making developments on speed, acceleration, fuel efficiency, and cornering. How competitive do you think that team would be?

That is the mindsight we're moving into. The 80/20 flip won't happen overnight, but it WILL happen. And once you come to believe that this is possible, everything else will start to slot into place.

Planning for The Start of Your 90 Days

Hopefully by now you are itching to get started. Your aim is nothing less than becoming the overall visionary of your organization, and that idea should excite and energize you.

Tech is the present AND the future of your healthcare organization, and no one is better placed to know what advancements are coming, and what the best solution is going to be to tackle current and future challenges. Therefore, you are the only one who has the ability to truly innovate.

One final mental exercise before we really get started. Ask yourself the following questions with a simple 'yes,' 'no,' or 'maybe.'

- In terms of upcoming tech purchases and developments, am I investigating the right options?

- Do I have the right processes in place to make good decisions regarding tech purchases or adaptations?

- Am I fulfilling compliance requirements, while still innovating for future growth?

- Do I have contingency plans for all of my departments and, if so, are those plans adequate?

- Am I meeting our customers' technology requirements now and, if so, do I have a plan to maintain this success?

- Am I vigorously managing our vendors in terms of their support, our contractual agreements, and the prices we're paying them?

- Is the money my organization is investing in IT making us more competitive?

O Am I taking responsibility for creating a competitive advantage?

O Am I keeping an eye on cutting-edge and disruptive technologies?

O Am I truly bringing value to the organization?

Don't worry if you're getting a lot, or even all, 'no's' and 'maybes.' If you were able to answer a resounding 'yes' to every question, you wouldn't need this book.

The point of this exercise is for you to get clear in your head what you're shooting for and where you can expect to be by the end of your evolution.

Or perhaps 'end' is the wrong word. Evolution never really ends, right?

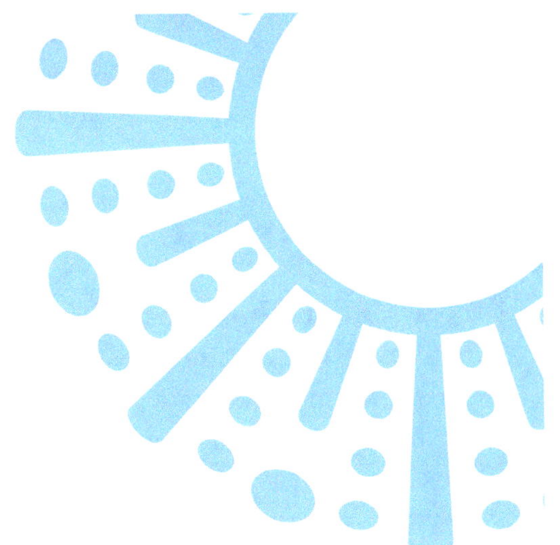

CHAPTER TWO

The 90-Day CIO Model: Going from Reactive to High Performance

Rodgers and Hammerstein tell us that the beginning is a very good place to start. In this instance I respectfully disagree. To become a high-performance CIO of a complex healthcare operation you're far better served by starting at the end and working backwards.

We're going to start by figuring out where we want you to be in 5-10 years, what needs to happen in that period to reach that end, and then what needs to happen in the next 90 days to start you on a journey that will reach that successful conclusion.

My aim for you is to eventually reach a position of high performance in which you add significant value to your organization, the patients and their families are happy, your staff are happy, and everything you manage has the gleam of excellence. But it is not like flipping a switch. You're not going to go from where you are now to the highest levels of achievement overnight. You're going to move through a number of discrete stages before you eventually reach your end goal.

Because every person and every organization are different, every journey is different, but it will look something like this…

Stage One: Reactive

Most CIOs and their departments, to a greater or lesser degree, tend to be fairly static, only spasming into life when a problem occurs. This is normal and is a legacy of developing during a period in which technology was limited and only had impact on 1-2 departments. Unfortunately, these practices are ill-suited to the modern world in which technology is the framework through which everything happens.

I have found that reactive healthcare organizations have the following characteristics:

- Federated departments with incompatible technology, creating walls between teams.

- Disparate processes for managing and maintaining the available technology.

- Inconsistent communication and management practices.

- Focus on short-term needs with little or no advance planning.

- Slow and cumbersome technology that frustrates the users.

- Minimal oversight and management of investments.

- Limited performance management of individuals.

- Low employee engagement and satisfaction scores.

Stage Two: Operational Excellence

By employing the strategies in this book, you will gradually attain the operational excellence stage. Teamwork and efficiency across all parts of the IT organization will be at an all-time high and most of the frustrations experienced by staff and patients will have been eliminated.

Healthcare organizations that have reached operational excellence have the following characteristics:

+ Clearly defined plans with a consistent IT operating model.

+ Common processes based on high standards.

+ Constant and clear communication and coordination between departments.

+ Consistently applied effective business and IT practices.

+ Good staff morale with above average engagement scores.

+ Best practices firmly embedded in all daily operations.

+ Operational and financial metrics clearly defined and achieved.

+ A model for transformational leadership.

+ Clear accountability across all levels of seniority.

Stage Three: High-Performance

Stage two might sound optimal, and there is no denying that it's a great feeling to reach this level of excellence. But there's another level to climb if you're going to truly maximize your organization's abilities.

High-performing healthcare organizations have the following characteristics:

+ Value for patients and their families, employees, and the organization as a whole established as the primary goal.

+ Anticipation of business needs across all departments.

+ High staff morale with high engagement scores.

+ Able to support coordinated care across the system.

+ Clinical systems that support the delivery of high quality, standardized care across the system.

+ A model of excellence at every level.

+ The creation of a learning organization that other businesses seek to learn from.

+ Improved quality across the board, with lowered costs wherever possible.

What is The Difference?

As an example, let's consider one of the core functions of the IT department: Helping staff and end-users resolve technical issues.

A **REACTIVE** organization, at its worst, will have no procedure for reporting and responding to support requests. Staff will simply grab a technician when they chance to pass one in a corridor and ask them to stop by when they get a chance. Or they'll have the extension number of the technician they get along with best on a post-it note stuck on their computer, and they'll call them up when their mouse stops working (hint: the batteries probably need changing). If the technician is on vacation, the staff member will simply live with the problem until they return.

If there are more technical problems than available staff, an ad hoc queue is created with priority generally given to the most senior person. Everyone else has to simply wait their turn. When a technical problem is tackled by an IT team member, regardless of whether they manage to resolve the issue, nothing is recorded in writing or digitally.

At its best, a centralized IT helpdesk number might be available with one or more operators standing by to take calls and route them to the best person who can help. But even in this, more organized scenario, this is still very much a reactive process. The IT team are order-takers – active when there's something to do and inactive when there isn't.

In contrast, an IT organization operating under **OPERATIONAL EXCELLENCE** will definitely have a standard helpdesk number or ticketing system that acts as the first port of call for a staff member needing technical support. But in addition, they will be operating under a "first call resolution" policy in which they attempt to resolve the problem straight away without the need to escalate the call to anyone else. A good target would be to reach a "first call resolution" rate of 90% or better.

In practice this can only happen if the helpdesk staff is using a service management system that advises them on how to fix most basic problems and they also adhere to the associated processes prescribed by the Information Technology Infrastructure Library (more on this in a future chapter).

If the problem is more complex, the helpdesk operator will advise the caller that their problem will be escalated to a programmer who will call them back. The call is important because a ticketing system, on its own, might not have sufficient information and then you have a situation where a solution is posited that is insufficient. A call also helps reassure the staff member that their problem has been registered and that a solution is being worked on.

Once a fix is found and the problem resolved, what happens next? The programmer documents the problem and how it was successfully resolved. They create a short article containing the details and add it to the helpdesk knowledgebase. So, now, the next time someone calls with a similar issue, the helpdesk person puts in the keywords, the article pops up, and this issue can be resolved during the first call, with no escalation required.

The longer this process is followed, the better the knowledgebase becomes, and the more support requests can be resolved on the first call. This is good for the caller who gets a quick resolution, good for the helpdesk responder who feels like they're performing a useful function (rather than just routing calls to more experienced team members all the time), and good for the more senior members of the IT team who aren't repeatedly being asked to fix the same problems over and over again. This means that they now have more time to perform more value-added functions.

This proactive element that ensures everything gets better and better for the end users with every interaction. It's what allows them to experience a real HELP DESK instead of just a call center.

A **HIGH PERFORMING** IT helpdesk moves things up a notch by aiming to help end users BEFORE a problem even occurs. It is all about anticipation. The IT leadership will review the incoming calls and the knowledgebase and look for trends. If the same problem is occurring in a lot of different departments, it might be that an underlying problem needs fixing that will stop this error occurring.

Or if it's a fairly simple issue that keeps cropping up in the same department, a high performing IT department might arrange a 30-minute training session with that particular team that either prevents the issue or shows them how to deal with it themselves.

Not only does this massively reduce end user downtime while significantly increasing their satisfaction levels, it frees up your IT team to work on long-term development projects without being constantly called away to put out little fires.

Moving from reactive to high-performing won't happen in 90 days, but at the end of the three months you'll be heading in that direction.

The Three Ages of The CIO

Some of my readers will look at the above and be daunted by the level of change I am promoting. Others will be energized by the challenge. Whichever camp you find yourself in, keep reminding yourself that this is a five, maybe even ten-year journey with hundreds of projects. No one should expect to make these transitions overnight.

So, for now, take a moment to review the characteristics of the final, high-performance stage and imagine how it will feel to reach this pinnacle. Allow yourself to taste the satisfaction and professional pride you're going to feel when you attain this level of sophistication. And remind yourself that this journey is essential for the evolution of your role and for the long-term survival of your healthcare organization. These three stages of organizational development are a mirror of the way in which the CIO role has changed.

The *first age* of the modern CIO harks back to the 1980s and 1990s which I like to think of as "The Plumber." The CIO in this age got the network up and running, got the emails going, put some services in place, and that was the bulk of the job.

The *second age* was in the early 2000s after the great Y2K efforts exhausted all of our energy and resources. This was when big tech budgets started being placed in the hands of the CIO, and they were tasked with fully digitizing the healthcare system and putting in shareable technology at the heart of every department. Many CIOs blossomed in this period, while others began to struggle and were replaced by more forward-thinking executives.

The *third age*, the one we're in now, is the era of innovation and the constant flow of digital information through Cloud services, mobile applications, and social networks. It's no longer enough for each department in a hospital to be connected; now the entire network of hospitals and care facilities need to be joined up 24 hours a day, 365 days a year.

This is where a CIO's ability to evolve has been tested to the limit. Being in the reactive stage was just about enough for the first age, but totally unsuited for the second age, and catastrophic for the third age. It's why CIOs that haven't updated their practices and methodologies are now finding themselves falling behind in terms of efficiencies, employee satisfaction, and patient outcomes.

That's the thing about "ages;" they only move forwards. Which means you have to move forward too.

The 90-Day CIO Model Framework

These days it seems that a good idea is worthless if you can't summarize it in under 10 words so that it can be understood by the lowest common denominator on the most superficial of levels. This wasn't something I aspired to do so instead I've created the next best thing – an image that encapsulates what your next 90 days are going to be about and what your priorities must be.

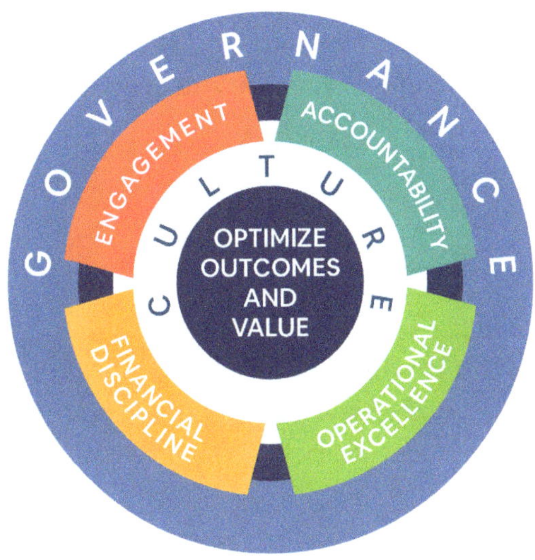

Figure 2.1. The 90 Day CIO Model ©

At the heart of this chart is the primary target of everything you're going to tackle in the next three months. Any time you find yourself floundering or lacking direction, remember that your end goal for the most part is to ***Optimize Patient Outcomes and Organizational Value***.

Accomplishing your goals can't be done through your own force of will, it has to be achieved by bringing your colleagues and your employees along for the ride. Which is why your primary goal is surrounded by the new ***Culture*** you're going to instigate.

On top of that culture you're going to build four key qualities that are going to come to epitomize your new strategy and your expectations for everyone you work with. Along with *Culture*, individual chapters are going to be spent discussing the critical importance of ***Accountability***, ***Financial Discipline***, ***Engagement***, and ***Operational Excellence***.

Last, but most certainly not least, your overarching efforts will lead to the establishment of solid ***Governance*** that will hold everything else together. If you put the pieces properly in place, in the long-term you should find yourself moving into a position where the majority of your time is spent keeping everyone and everything within the guidelines you create, and leading by example.

IT Triple Aim

The above is the simplest way in which I can explain the 90-Day CIO Model. But it is only a summary. And while I hope it is useful in helping you stay clear on what you are trying to achieve at each step, it is of course necessary to expand on what your overall goals will be.

Let's begin by reviewing the triple aim of healthcare which will also become the beacon for us in the IT organization:

✦ Better Health

✦ Better Care

✦ Lower Costs

Much of what I cover in the rest of the book contains varying degrees of discretion that you will likely adapt and adjust depending on the unique needs of your healthcare organization. The triple aim of healthcare and of the IT organization however does not. They are non-negotiable. Each is critical and none can be excluded or minimized without hindering your ability to become the CIO of a high-performing healthcare network.

Better Health belongs at the top of the list because making the patients feel better physically, mentally and emotionally is the first calling of all healthcare professionals, including those of us in IT.

Better Care closely follows it because once we've cared for the health of our patients, they should also feel as if they've been treated with respect and dignity, and that they've been cared for as an individual who deserves to be treated like the important human being they are.

Lower Costs completes the trilogy because modern healthcare also needs to be profitable. As is often said "no money no mission." While your direct impact on the overall profitability of the organization may seem somewhat limited, you can contribute significantly by looking for ways to reduce costs and wastage, without negatively impacting the high standards you're establishing.

Your first task then, in the 90-Day CIO Strategy is to take the above chart, as well as the triple aim, and put it in a place where you can see it every day, multiple times a day. You could pin it to the wall of your office. You could write it on post-it notes and stick it on your desk. You could make it the lock screen image on your phone. Or you could do all the above.

I also urge you to share this information with everyone you speak with over the next 90 days about this journey so they're also clear on your personal goals and therefore your expectations for them.

It's up to you how you want to put these concepts front and center in your mind, but I encourage you to do something to this end.

If you want to put this book down and go ahead and carry out this exercise now, feel free to do so. Alternatively, if you prefer to finish reading each section before taking action, you'll find a helpful summary of the recommended steps at the end of each chapter.

IT Guiding Principles

Your next step is to create a list of your IT guiding principles. You may already have something along these lines, in which case now is a good time to review and update it.

This is the first example of a recommendation that needs to be tailored to the individual requirements of your organization so I can't give you a standard list. I can, however, give you the list that I have personally successfully used during my consulting and CIO roles at multiple healthcare systems throughout the country. Feel free to borrow it, adapt it, or steal it outright.

- Commitment to quality, patient safety, and coordinated care.

- Timely, definitive, inclusive decision-making.

- Collaborative and creative problem-solving.

- Frequent, targeted, and accurate communications,

- Integrated systems and standardized processes.

- Well-planned, efficient implementations.

- Put the patient first in all decisions.

- Create an information technology environment that will encourage patients to prefer our organization.

- Enable consistent, evidence-based standards of excellence across all venues of care.

- Enable the provision of the most personalized and coordinated care across all venues.

- Deliver all the information needed by providers and staff to make the proper care decisions.

- Facilitate the engagement of patients and their families actively and effectively in their care.

- Plan our work and hold ourselves accountable to aggressive but achievable milestones and performance metrics, including financials.

- Be creative in the development of learning materials to ensure efficient, scenario-based training and quick end-user adoption.

- Commit to strict quality assurance and adhering to defined testing, data migration, and software change processes.

Set Your Five (or Ten) Year Targets

Once you have your list of guiding principles – which, by the way, can be adjusted or added to over the coming months as your understanding of the project develops – you can turn these into more tangible targets and prioritize accordingly.

For example, if one of your goals is to put the patient first in all decisions, what might this look like in practice? Are you going to create or modify standard operating procedures for how a patient's needs and preferences are extracted and recorded? Are you going to create a training program for patient-facing staff that helps them improve in this area? Are you going to bring in a consultant to review your existing practices?

Make a list of ideas for every principle in your list and engage others in putting them in order of priority. You don't have to commit to everything you write down and, in practice, this list is going to change multiple times over the coming months and years. Think of it more as a chance to imagine what you want your department to look like once you've reached the high-performing stage, and what positive changes you could make to get you there.

Sharpen Your Ax

There's an old saying – usually incorrectly attributed to Abraham Lincoln – that if you're going to cut down a tree in five minutes, you should spend three minutes sharpening your ax. Adapting this to our journey, if you're going to create a high-performing healthcare organization in the next 5-10 years, you need to spend 90 days putting things in motion.

Realistically you're not going to be able to accomplish everything that needs to be done on your own. Once you have your plans in place, you need to get your colleagues on board and show them how to start rolling out the changes on which you're going to insist.

All the projects below are covered in more detail in future chapters, but you should find it helpful to review what you have to look forward to so you can prepare yourself for the challenges ahead.

Create Executive Performance in Yourself

You cannot lead others until you're confidently and effectively managing yourself with precision. You must, at every step of the way, lead by example and be prepared to work with people to help them understand what you're creating and why it's so important. You may find this stage a breeze or it may take considerable effort.

Establish Your Position in The Leadership Team Externally and Internally

If the people you work most closely with are not fully aware with what your role entails, you can be sure that the people and departments with whom you have limited contact are also in the dark. You are going to change this in the most effective way possible by meeting and talking regularly with everyone whose lives you are going to impact either individually or at the very least in a group.

Enhance Your Culture with Superior Communication and Engagement

The chapter in this book on the subject of culture might just be the most important of all. You can set up and train people in the most amazing and effective strategies imaginable, but culture will prevent anyone from adopting it if it doesn't mesh with "how things have always been done." Creating a new culture that embraces high performance is going to be one of the most valuable and far-reaching projects you ever complete for your organization.

Create Financial and Contractual Discipline

This is one of those projects that sounds nebulous but actually involves very specific procedures that people are going to follow when it comes to selecting and integrating new tech. The result is going to be not a new era of penny-pinching and redundancies, but a paradigm that allows people to have a direct say in the tech they're going to use and a budget with which to do it.

Turn Vendors into Partnerships

You're, no doubt, dependent on many vendors to supply and manage various parts of your technology infrastructure. And you're going to continue to do so. But you're also going to reposition things so that, instead of it being a pseudo parent-and-child relationship, you're going to become partners. Your successes are going to be their successes and vice-versa.

Organizational Structures Changed to Improve The Whole

Communication, best practices, and management structures will almost certainly need to change to create the kind of nimble, transparent processes you need to cope with modern technological challenges. In some cases this may mean giving more authority to some individuals. In other cases it might mean positioning team members in more than one department.

Identify and Assign Governance Committees

Gaining control of decision-making processes doesn't mean adding layers of needless bureaucracy or setting yourself up as a grand administrator who has to approve every decision. Governance committees, when structured correctly, can actually speed up decision-making and give individuals more ownership of the projects they're working on. At the same time, you're going to identify and nail down the most critical decision-making steps so you can keep a firm hand on expenditure.

Operational Excellence Using ITIL

Your Information Technology Infrastructure Library (ITIL) is key to the efficacy of your IT administrators and support team. Unless you've already done so in the last 12 months, you're long overdue for a full review and refresh.

Cybersecurity Stress Testing

This could be an entire book on its own, which is why it at least warrants its own chapter. Your focus, especially within the first 90 days, is not the technical aspects of cybersecurity (which is constantly changing anyway) but rather the human element. Accountability across your entire team is crucial and you will be creating mock phishing exercises to ensure there are no weak links.

Schedule Regular Meetings

Daily, weekly, monthly, quarterly and annual meetings can be optimized to ensure you don't lose the bulk of your time to idle chat, while at the same time ensuring that you keep abreast of everything that's happening in terms of IT, and that every member of the staff feels involved and listened to.

Review Your Plans with The Leadership

None of your plans are going to come to fruition unless every last person is willing to work with you. Not because you rule with an iron fist, but because they firmly believe in what you're trying to achieve and they recognize the future benefits to themselves, their colleagues, and the patients.

Scheduling Your 90 Days

This is just a taste of what's to come, but you can already start to think about how you want to ration out your 90 days. Again, I cannot give you a one-size-fits-all because a lot is going to depend on what you already have in place or what may need building from scratch.

Provisionally, you might consider something along the lines of…

- ✦ 1-30 Days: Assessment Month (reviewing existing collateral and speaking with your colleagues and employees.)

- ✦ 30-60 Days: Planned Development Month (finalizing the structural changes you intend to make, as well as new procedures.)

- ✦ 60-90 Days: Execution Month (instructing your team to carry out the planned developments and monitoring their progress.)

To-Do List: Part One
(Your 90-Day CIO Strategy Overview)

☐   **Task #1** – Place the 90-Day CIO Strategy and the IT Triple Aim somewhere where you will see it multiple times a day. Regularly review it so that your primary targets become burned into your brain. Look for opportunities, also, to share these with your colleagues.

☐   **Task #2** – Create (or review) your IT guiding principles. Update it based on your developing understanding of what a high-performing healthcare organization looks like.

☐   **Task #3** – Set your five (or ten) year targets based on what you need to achieve and then use these to brainstorm a list of tangible milestones. With the engagement and assistance of others, arrange these targets and milestones in order of priority.

☐   **Task #4** – Put together a rough schedule for the next 90 days that allows room for reviewing, planning, and then executing your plans.

How Bad Can It Be?

Do not be alarmed if you've recently landed a new CIO position and you've inherited an organization that's very much stuck in the reactive stage. Even the bleakest of scenarios can be turned around using the 90-day method.

In one of my previous roles (that I won't name out of respect for the fine people I worked with there), the organization was a couple of decades behind on best practices. One of the first things I noticed when I was finding my way around the departments was that my assistant had these big piles of papers stacked on her desk. I asked her what they were for, and she explained that every night the data center operator printed out reports for all the different departments so that, the following morning, someone from each team could stop by and collect them.

This was shocking to me. It was a waste of paper (since I was fairly certain many of the reports would end up being tossed without even being read), it was a waste of this intelligent lady and operator's time, and it was staggeringly inefficient. This was the kind of process we phased out back in the '90s before we had printers distributed throughout the organization. Why wasn't everyone logging onto their applications and downloading their own reports?

Less than a month into my role I visited each department head and explained that we weren't going to be centrally printing reports anymore. If they needed the information they could log-in to their application and print what they needed (and only what they needed) directly. It would be easier, faster, and less wasteful of everyone's precious time. Unanimously, they all agreed.

The exercise did not take long, but in one fell swoop, and only a few weeks into the job, I had already helped to improve the efficiency of the organization and the leadership knew that I was going to be focused on modernizing the organization and driving out inefficiencies.

Other Challenges Took Longer to Resolve.

For example, when it came to promotions, there was very much a "time served" policy in operation. Whoever had sat in their seat the longest expected to get the job, regardless of whether their skills and experience made them a good fit. This was not an insignificant problem. Very early on I had a position to fill and the person in line was totally unsuited for the role. And, unlike the above problem, I couldn't simply change the rules. There was a union to take into consideration, and putting my foot down and refusing to give the role to the expected person would have created considerable problems. Frankly, I wanted to keep my powder dry for bigger issues.

But that didn't mean the situation was hopeless. I sat down with the person in line for the position, described what they would be required to do in the role and what I would expect from them on a daily basis. And then asked the question: "Are you confident that you can do all of that?" Fortunately, the individual was honest enough to say "no" and he turned down the position, leaving me free to select the right person.

To tackle a resolutely reactive organization, sometimes you need to find some creative responses. What you can't do is just let things slide and hope that everyone will move towards a high-performance level if you simply set a good example. You're going to have to *make* things happen.

The biggest challenge was getting my IT team engaged in their work. Their culture was unrelentingly doing what was required and asked of them, and not one iota more.

We start at 8. We leave at 3. We get our break at 10:30. As long as the lights stay on, we've achieved our goals.

That was the mindset I was dealing with and, to be honest, I'd never experienced such low levels of engagement. I could shoot a cannon down the IT department at 4:30pm and never be in any danger of hitting anyone (ignore the rumors, I never actually did this). It's hard to imagine a more precise example of a reactive organization.

Resolving those issues took time (the methods described in the upcoming chapter on culture were particularly useful) but eventually we got closer to the kind of well-coordinated, well-planned team that I was used to working with and that I always demand from the departments I lead.

So, if your situation right now looks bleak, take heart. Work the 90-day plan and by the end you'll have a firm foundation on which to eventually construct a strong, high-performing healthcare organization.

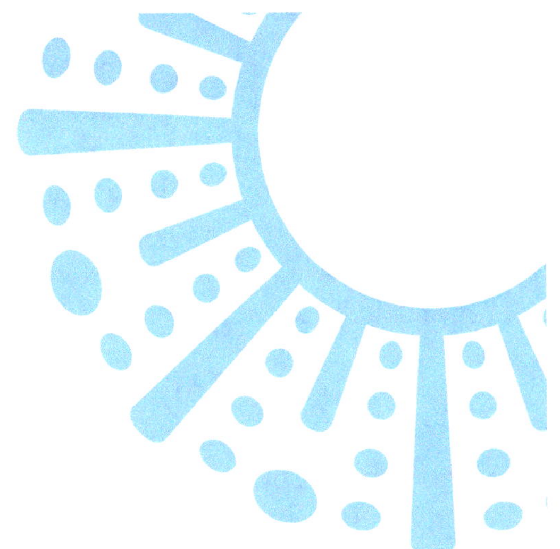

CHAPTER THREE:

Focus – Optimize Patient Outcomes and Organizational Value

As you read this book you may be asking yourself "what's the problem we're trying to solve?" Well, the problem is that a lot of hospital executives, including CIOs, care too much. And, no, that's not intended as a compliment. Let me explain.

Let's start by looking at the Triple Aim again, but this time think of it as being listed in order of priority.

+ Better Health

+ Better Care

+ Lower Costs

Why is "Health" more important than "Care?" Because caring can only get you so far. In fact, I believe that many healthcare organizations could serve their patients' health better by focusing a little less on care and a little more on management. If that sounds cold, it's only because we've come to associate management with business and profit and corporate sensibilities. When in fact "manage" simply means to be in charge.

This is a crucial difference because you can only care for your patients directly while they're in your facilities. And your goal is to keep patients, by virtue of improved health, out of your facilities as much as possible. It's better for your patients and it's better for your resources.

It's like the old joke about the man who says he trusts his mechanic absolutely, which is why he takes his car to the garage every week. If our patients keep coming back to us it might be because they trust our healthcare services. But it might equally be because we haven't done enough to prevent the recurrence or progression of their ailments.

In short, it's all too easy to give patients what we feel we can reasonably give them under the circumstances, rather than what they actually need. Whereas if we took a long-term, and a truly holistic, view of a person's health, we would quickly realize that the very manner in which our organization is arranged is totally ill-suited to create the best possible outcomes for our patients and indeed their families. The fact is that despite all of our efforts, we're still a sick care instead of the true healthcare system that we know we need to be. Our education, infrastructure and processes are still focused on treating patients when they are sick and not on keeping them well. Our compensation and other incentives systems are still continuing to drive specialization and not generalization without an equal focus on prevention and treatment. Accountable care can solve this, but in the meantime, we need to continue to do what is best while minding the gaps the incentives create. I don't mean this as a criticism of our system but more as a statement of the facts that need to be considered as we contemplate how we're going to truly impact the health and wellness of our patients and their families.

But quick, let us change the subject. Because if we really think about how badly we're failing our patients we might feel compelled to do something about it. And that is a daunting prospect. It feels impossible. Far better to close this book and focus on something you can fix, like improving the ticketing system for your IT support desk.

No, of course you are better than that. You're reading this book because you know in your heart that there's a better way. And as the person at the forefront of the technology and processes that can genuinely improve patient and family outcomes, you have an awesome opportunity to make a difference in the lives of tens, maybe hundreds, of thousands of people.

Tear Down The Walls

Hospital departments have a reputation for not communicating efficiently with each other. The goals aren't aligned, the technology being used may be different and incompatible, and everyone's too busy to seriously collaborate. If that's true of hospital departments, it's even more true of different clinics and facilities within a wider healthcare network.

But people downplay this problem because everything still kind of works. Patients get moved from one specialist to the next, and their medical records mostly follow. And even though nothing is as quick and efficient as it could be, it's working well enough to keep things ticking along.

This is the first notion of which you need to disabuse yourself. And, in time, you need to convince everyone around you of this as well. The silos that departments operate within create walls between colleagues, and the results are far worse than mere inefficiency. Insufficient communication can result in poor quality treatment, and, to compound matters, the impact and cause can also itself be incorrectly communicated.

Imagine, for instance, a patient recovering from a heart attack who is encouraged to go for daily walks. However, because of poor communication, the physician is unaware that the patient is going through a bereavement and, as a result, has become mildly agoraphobic. How likely is it that the recommended daily exercise is actually going to happen? When the second heart attack inevitably happens, this is recorded as a relapse with no recognition that this could potentially have been avoided if the patient's limitations had been considered.

Or how about the chronic depressive who is referred to a local therapy group by a family doctor, but because of limited access to previous appointment notes, they miss the fact that the patient is also arthritic and lives on the third floor of a building in which the elevator is broken. The depression escalates into self-harm, but no one registers that this could have been avoided if better communication had taken place.

Even worse, there's the young man who is prescribed antimalarial tablets for his trip to the Caribbean, but because digital medical records aren't correctly aligned, no one notices that this will clash with his existing medication, resulting in a dangerous arrhythmia. A local doctor recognizes the problem and advises the patient to stop taking the antimalarial tablets. The patient assumes it's a simple side-effect, chalks it down to experience, and the conflicting medication issue is not reported or tackled.

But surely, you might ask, with finite time and resources, there is only so much that can be done to treat the patient in a truly holistic manner? Aren't we in danger of extending our reach beyond what is feasible?

Simply... no. In fact, I think we should go even further and start factoring in social determinants.

In the unlikely event that you're not familiar with them, social determinants are non-medical contributors to a person's health (or lack thereof). It's estimated that these factors account for as much as 55% of a person's overall health which potentially places it higher on the list of determinants than healthcare or even lifestyle. According to the World Health Organization, examples include…

- Income and social protection

- Education

- Unemployment and job insecurity

- Working life conditions

- Food insecurity

- Housing, basic amenities and the environment

- Early childhood development

- Social inclusion and non-discrimination

- Structural conflict

- Access to affordable health services of decent quality.

When considering the most appropriate treatment for the patients that your healthcare organization looks after, how many of those factors are considered on a regular basis?

Well, while I'm stressing you out, let's add another social determinant: family circumstances. Do they live alone? Do they have dependents? Do they have other family members in poor health?

Remember, the first half of the title of this chapter is optimizing patient outcomes. I believe that there are really no limits on how far we should be prepared to go to assess the patients we care for, individually, but also as a group. Understanding the communities that live in your catchment area should be seen as fundamental to delivering long-term, successful outcomes for everybody.

Believe me when I tell you, no matter how impossible such a challenge may seem, it is not only possible, but also necessary. And it starts by tearing down the walls between your departments and improving your technology (and the methodologies for using and managing them) so that communication is clear, consistent and effective.

Instead of being a collection of disparate teams each with their own culture, objectives and methods, you're going to transition into a single team with everybody pulling together to reach the same end goal: better healthcare outcomes for patients and their families.

This isn't something you can do on your own. And it certainly isn't something you can do if the people you manage are not on the same page with each other and don't understand or share your vision. Getting everyone to embrace your quest and pursue it relentlessly is going to be one of the most important tasks you complete during these first 90 days, and we'll discuss methods for accomplishing this in the next chapter.

For now, grab your notepad and start making some notes. Make a list of the data you need and where you can obtain it. It might be department heads, it might be community leaders, it might be the police, it might be housing associations, even the fire service. You're going to have to think creatively, and it may be that some of the data you need doesn't exist in a form currently available to you. You might need to create a method for gathering it.

Write it all down. Get it out of your head and onto the page.

Once you are done, give some thought to how you're going to analyze and assess the data once you have it. Is this a role that you are well-suited for? If not, who do you need to draft into this project to help you?

Do Not Get Hung Up on The Details

If you're of a certain personality type, you might immediately start to see the problems and pitfalls. And if you're not careful you might quickly reach the conclusion that what you're attempting to do is unrealistic and probably futile. It's not and it isn't, and that's why we call them "knee jerk reactions."

This isn't going to be easy, but I've done this enough times to know that this exercise is very effective and is by no means impossible.

In economics there is a concept called "Perfect Information" in which analysts assume that everyone has a perfect understanding and complete knowledge of everything in their model. Of course, in practice it isn't always possible to gather every piece of information, and some information may ultimately be unavailable to you. But that doesn't mean you abandon the project or keep trying to gather data until you have every last possible crumb (an endless and futile goal). Instead, you look past the limitations and draw conclusions on what you have and the parts of the data that seem to be most germane.

Ultimately you will likely find that this exercise is simpler than you think. There's a very good chance that there's a department or organization out there that already has the bulk of the information you need; more than enough for you to be able to draw useful conclusions about the community you serve. It's simply a matter of finding them and working with them.

Collaboration is the key to all of this.

I once had a meeting in which the chief nursing officer was reporting troubling information about how short-staffed they were. Then, in the very next meeting I attended, the CFO recommended cutting some of our nursing staff so we could hit our financial goals.

This is what happens when departments are misaligned and not communicating effectively. You're going to tackle this head-on and start a new era of transparency and real teamwork.

Embrace Population Health Management

For the uninitiated, Population Health Management (PHM) is a strategy that aims to improve the physical and mental health of a community by focusing on things other than access to health care. Primarily, this means looking at the kinds of social determinants discussed earlier in this chapter. A basic example would be improving housing that is damp and cold and that might later create respiratory problems in the inhabitants.

Crucially, PHM does not wait until people get sick before making efforts to help them. A well-integrated system can identify at risk individuals and offer support now that might reduce the risk of serious health problems later on. For instance, a doctor with access to the right data and the time and resources to research their patients, might identify individuals at high risk of diabetes or heart attack, and proactively reach out to them for a discussion about helpful lifestyle changes.

At its peak, PHM can reduce duplication of efforts and significantly shorten waiting lists and reduce time-to-care. This is better for the patients and their families, naturally, but is also better for the healthcare providers in terms of reduced stress and improved job satisfaction.

If you already have a PHM program in your organization or area, a lot of the hard work may have already been done for you. If so, get involved. Find out what resources and initiatives are already available that can be introduced to your healthcare organization. But also, consider what you can do to further support and expand the program. For example, some PHM initiatives have used virtual consultations to allow patients to meet with multiple specialists simultaneously. You can, no doubt, appreciate how potentially beneficial this is to help the individual receive a joined-up treatment plan.

If you don't have a PHM program in your area, you could be a catalyst to initiate one. If that isn't feasible, at the very least you should be familiar with the different elements of PHM and consider how you might be able to influence the introduction of these initiatives into your organization.

PHM: Care Integration

This is one of the broadest elements of PHM that seeks to link up social needs and healthcare needs. At its most basic level, for instance, this might involve giving patients at your healthcare facilities access to healthcare advice at housing association offices. At one of the organizations I worked in, we made great strides to reach out to those who had limited access to healthcare services, either by choice or by circumstance, by visiting barber shops and salons on the weekends. We brought our mobile healthcare services to these locations because we knew that these people in need frequented them on the weekends. The idea is to identify the intersection between peoples' health and social needs and allow related organizations to combine their efforts to reach them.

More targeted opportunities also exist. For example, patients with type-2 diabetes could be assessed to identify those who are also at risk of developing depression and anxiety. A proactive program could contact these patients, educate them on the link between their physical and mental health, and make them aware of services that can support them.

We can only scratch the surface here. And while you should definitely brainstorm this topic, you'll likely gain far more ideas by talking to your colleagues and team members. You may be surprised how many of them already have ideas that they assume no one would ever take the time to seriously consider.

PHM: Care Coordination

This can be summarized as efficiency in supporting patients to ensure time and resources are not wasted. It starts by identifying patients who are considered high-risk, sharing information with related departments, and managing each patient's use of the care available to them.

Identifiers for people who would benefit from this kind of support might include:

- Patients with multiple conditions.

- Patients with long-term chronic illnesses.

- Patients who have made repeated inappropriate visits to ER.

- Patients on a wide variety of medications that have not been recently reviewed.

- Patients receiving unusually expensive levels of care.

Assisting these people could be achieved by discussing their cases with the different departments they're connected with, providing them with a Care Coordinator who takes responsibility for liaising with them to ensure they're getting the most appropriate care, or simply creating better systems and processes for following-up after procedures or tests.

PHM: Teamwork

The age of individual specialists working with patients on an individual basis has gone. It cannot be overstated how important it is for specialists, nurses, care managers, pharmacists, counsellors, and resource coordinators to have a method by which they can share information clearly and easily, and actually talk to each other about the care being provided.

It is also important to recognize the pivotal role that nurses play across the whole spectrum of care. More than any other care givers, nurses are well-placed to understand the unique needs of each individual. Involving nurses in the construction of new, team-based systems, and providing them with training to take advantage of the tools and resources you're going to make available to them is going to be key. More than likely, they will be your most critical end-users.

PHM: Patient Engagement

The phrases, PHM and Patient Engagement, are often used interchangeably, but they are not really the same thing. While PHM focuses on non-healthcare factors that can be addressed to improve overall health outcomes, Patient Engagement refers to directly engaging individuals in actions that will improve their own health.

So, while a PHM initiative might involve, for instance, improving housing conditions, this is something that is out of the hands of the individuals who benefit. A Patient Engagement initiative, however, might for example invite individuals to take part in exercise programs that reduce their risk of heart disease and stroke. Other examples could include diet support groups, healthy cooking workshops, exercise routines, nature walks, and so on. From the technology side, you may want to consider using the connected smart televisions that are starting to proliferate our patient's home to engage them in complying with their medication regimens or to let them know about the pollen count in their neighborhood that morning.

The key is to empower individuals with information and services to help them to take responsibility for improving their health prospects and recognize the ability they have to improve their long-term prospects.

PHM: Data Analytics and Health Information Technology

With your responsibility and expertise in technology and your efforts to continuously provide better and more innovative solutions, data analytics is going to be your bread and butter when it comes to PHM. We have data available to us on a magnitude beyond anything previously imagined and we now have the tools to help us analyze and interpret it.

Whereas data might once have been limited to age, gender, address, and insurance, now we have a myriad of readily available information including family history, genetic factors, and environmental risks. And with the rapid rise in popularity of wearables, we can also start to factor in lifestyle factors such as sleep quality, mobility, heart rates, and much more.

Ultimately this is what will allow your healthcare organization to move a long way from a one-size-fits-all approach and instead offer an individual service, tailored to each patient's specific needs.

PHM: Value-based Care

For now, this is outside the scope of this book, but value-based care – in which healthcare organizations are reimbursed based on patient outcomes rather than services rendered – is going to become increasingly the norm for patient populations. This may or may not be something you welcome, but what is certain is that PHM is going to be one of your best tools for operating under this arrangement.

PHM, by design, affords you the opportunity to consider behavioral health issues, non-clinical risk factors, and social and economic conditions. Basically, all the things that will allow you to make a success of value-based care. Factor in PHM's focus on prevention and you have a perfect synergy that should allow you to provide the infrastructure and applications that make this an overwhelmingly financial success of this arrangement.

Going Beyond Your Role

In one of my previous CIO roles, we had two Accountable Care Organizations (ACOs) in operation. You're likely familiar with this, but just in case, an ACO is a coordinated group of healthcare providers working together, with the goal of providing better overall care to patients by reducing errors and duplicated efforts. Incentives are also provided to produce better overall results which helps drive initiatives for proactive programs. For instance, one of the methods the government used to improve quality and drive down costs was to assign groups of Medicare patients to specific doctors or to a specific ACO, rather than allow people to choose their physician. Less choice for the patient, but more opportunities for the healthcare organizations to proactively manage people's ongoing health challenges.

At this particular organization we had two ACOs, and from an operational standpoint they weren't operating with any real efficacy. The strategic planning just was not there. So, I sat down with the medical staff and the administrative staff at the ACO and we began to make a plan. Here's an example of some of the goals we put in place:

+ To put the beneficiary and family at the center of all its activities. It will honor individual preferences and engage people in shared decision-making.

+ To ensure coordination of care for beneficiaries regardless of its time or place.

+ To attend carefully to care transitions, especially as beneficiaries journey from one part of the care system to another.

+ To manage resources carefully and respectfully, make investments where necessary, and move resources to meet beneficiaries' needs.

+ To continually reduce its dependence on inpatient care.

+ To be proactive by reaching out to patients with reminders and advice that can help them stay healthy and let them know when it is time for a checkup or a test.

+ To collect, evaluate, and use data on healthcare processes sufficiently to measure what it achieves for beneficiaries and communities over time and use such data to improve care delivery and patient outcomes.

+ To be innovative in the service of the three-part aim of better care for individuals, better health for populations, and lower growth in expenditures.

+ To invest in the development and pride of its own workforce, including clinicians.

Ultimately, we spent two full days at a retreat, and we came up with a plan to tackle some of the medical challenges where we could make the most difference. We looked at cardiac and cancer patients, but the biggest focus was on a disease that affected a significant portion of the population: Diabetes. This was an ideal challenge to take on, because treatment and management is complex, with a lot of moving parts, and a lot of different specialists involved. Additionally, when diabetes is not treated properly, it leads to serious complications that are expensive to resolve and can result in life-changing disabilities. In terms of the Triple Aim (better health, better care, lower costs) we discussed in the previous chapter, this was an ideal target for quickly improving the outcomes for a large percentage of our patients.

I started out by speaking to the primary care physicians and discovering how they currently managed patients, what kinds of issues they had, and what they would like to see changed that they believed would improve the outcomes. For instance, one of the things we kept hearing was that they had too many people to see in too short a space of time. So, a proposed solution was to task the nurses with performing some of the steps that the physicians were currently managing.

These consultations and research were carried out before the retreat so that, once we had everyone together for the two days, I already had a lot of the key information, but also, I had input from the people who would be putting these strategies into practice. I saw myself as guiding the process but allowing the people on the front line the opportunity to drive the discussion and decide on the plans of action. At the end of the day, *they* were going to be the ones who had to implement whatever we agreed, so they needed to have ownership of the new strategy and have belief in it. I wasn't there to prescribe the end results; I was there to work with them and help them come up with the best plan.

The solution we landed on was to use the hemoglobin A1C scale to risk stratify patients, and then put together a coordinated plan to try to move people into a lower risk category. So, for example, the patients who had an A1C score of seven and above – already diabetic – would get proactive calls from their primary care physician's office to make sure they had the resources they needed to eat the right kinds of food and engage in some kind of exercise, that they had their eyes and feet examined every year, that they were properly keeping track of their blood sugar levels, and so on. In the same vein, the people whose A1C level was at six - pre-diabetic - would get proactive guidance to help them move down into the non-risk category.

This is classic population health management strategy and it's highly effective. As a result of this type of rigorous management of our patients, our ACOs experienced great results in both outcomes and cost which was beneficial to the patients and those who cared for them.

If you're sharp, you may have thought to ask the question: Why is a CIO getting involved in the management and operation of ACOs? Because, yes, this was technically beyond my role. But I saw the value in proposing and then managing these exercises because, first, it brought value to the overall organization; and there's nothing wrong with going that extra mile to improve something that it is within your power to improve. And second, because I was able to bring an IT perspective to an area that didn't, at the time, have mature solutions. My involvement afforded me the opportunity to observe the current and future IT needs of the ACOs and start to build solutions that would support their efforts.

We'll talk more in future chapters about getting involved in existing operations and committees so you can bring IT benefits to different areas, but for now I simply want you to appreciate the benefits of being proactive in your CIO position. This is a key part of how you go from being a reactive organization to a high-performing organization.

To-Do List: Part Two
(Your 90-Day CIO Strategy Overview)

☐　**Task #1** – Write out a list of the social determinants that you believe to be most relevant to the community you care for.

☐　**Task #2** – Arrange to speak to other department heads within your organization who may be able to provide additional insights in this area.

☐　**Task #3** – Widen the scope and reach out to organizations and community leaders who may also be able to provide useful insights and recommendations.

☐　**Task #4** – Once you have a good overall view of the social determinants for your region, consider the data that will help you gain a deeper understanding, the organizations that can help you obtain this data, and the person or persons inside or outside of your organization who can help you and the rest of the leadership team interpret this data and turn it into valuable information for all.

☐　**Task #5** – If you have a PHM program in your organization or area, contact those responsible and inquire as to how you can support them more fully and even expand their reach. If you do not have a PHM program in your area, speak to people within your organization to make your own list of potential initiatives you could create on your own or assist in creating.

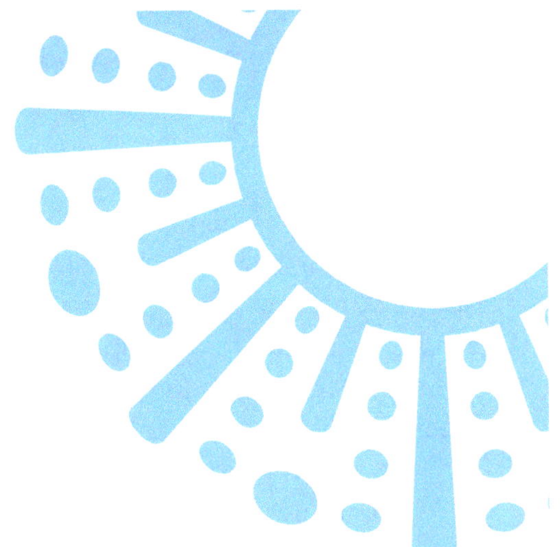

CHAPTER FOUR:

Culture – Creating the Foundation of Communication and Trust

It can't be reasoned with. It doesn't feel pity, or remorse, or fear. And it absolutely will not stop... ever.

No, I am not talking about the killer robot from the classic 1984 movie. I'm talking about the omnipresent force that pervades every part of every society that exists, that has ever existed, and that ever will exist: Culture.

We tend to think of culture in terms of a country's dress code and dining and music, but actually culture exists at every level of society and manifests itself in a wealth of small behaviors and attitudes. Every state in America has its own culture. Every city has its own unique nuances. Every school. Every office building. Every family.

Lock two people in a room and within a matter of days those two different personalities will have combined to develop their own simple culture.

Because when we talk about culture, at its most basic level, we are talking about ideas, customs and social behaviors that persist. And as long as at least one person exists in a single place or routine, a culture is going to develop. You can't stop it from happening, and although it can be changed and modified through external pressures, when the dust settles a culture will always develop.

Culture can be immensely valuable in the workplace because it gives employees a sense of comfort and familiarity. A feeling that they know how things work and that they can work within the cultural constructs to get things done. However, culture can also be detrimental. Behaviors can develop in a team of employees that are negative, or at the very least stultifying, such as a reluctance to volunteer for important tasks or a stamping out of original thoughts and ideas. Once negative attitudes exist in a culture, it can be very hard to counter them.

Additional challenges occur when two cultures clash, something commonly seen when two departments or even businesses merge. When two groups of disparate people and practices combine, a new culture will eventually emerge, but before then there will be arguments, tears, and likely even some turnover of staff.

Underestimate Culture at Your Peril

I've been told over and over again in academic and business circles that culture will eat strategy for lunch any day and I have experienced that in spades.

Some years ago, I was engaged by a large multi-hospital system to assist them in consolidating several data centers. The goal was to reduce everything down to just two centers that would back each other up. My team and I had helped many organizations with similar projects, some in far more complex environments, so this should have been a walk in the park.

But it was not.

We worked with the client leadership team to develop an extensive strategy and a detailed implementation plan for migrating all of the clinical and administrative applications in a seamless fashion. The idea was to complete the migration swiftly and efficiently, and in a way that would not result in outages for end-users. Essentially, we gave them a step-by-step plan for getting the job done.

Yet after a number of quarterly meetings, it became clear that very little progress was being made. As one of the leading partners on the project, and the one responsible for quality assurance, I met with the client's leadership regularly. And while they were friendly and engaging, even enthusiastic about the project, there was clearly something holding things back.

After many frustrating months I concluded that the problem was, of course, the client's organizational culture. They were lacking clear communication, basic coordination, and most importantly accountability. For example, I typically train my teams to be accepting of mistakes and to respond by creating and presenting a corrective plan. By contrast, this organization was more inclined to overlook or even obscure failure.

On top of these problems, there was a strong suspicion that the leadership members on the project were more focused on planning their retirement than making this crucial data centers consolidation happen.

Eventually I went into a meeting with the lead executive on their team and wrote on a piece of paper three major milestones that needed to be accomplished. I put the paper in an envelope and placed it on top of a large credenza in his office. I explained that if those three milestones were not met within the next six months, I would pull my team from the project.

With hindsight I think they thought I was bluffing. This was a very lucrative contract for me, and my partners and I believe there was a certain assumption that we weren't serious about walking away. Needless to say that after six months, I reviewed the three milestones and not a single one had been completed. We walked away, frustrated, from what was a multi-million-dollar engagement.

And while there was little else we could have done to salvage the project, the fact remains that this was a clear example of culture eating OUR strategy for lunch. If we'd kept going it would have also eaten our dinner, our dessert, and probably the brandy and cigars as well.

The good news, of course, is that you're not an external consultant. You're the CIO of your healthcare organization and, as such, you have the time, the access, and the resources to study the culture of your departments and mold it into something perfectly suited to your long-term plans.

Because although culture will naturally develop and eventually solidify on its own, top-down pressure can absolutely change an existing cultural environment. It'll take more than a few workshops and memos – these will do little more than move the needle slightly before everything springs back to the way things have always been – but with the right approach, you can massage the culture of your departments into something with strong, clear communication, well-coordinated methodologies, and accountability at every level. Everything that wasn't present in the example above.

How confident am I in the ability of management to shape a new culture? Confident enough that having accomplished it many times over in the workplace, I'm now seeking to change the culture of an entire industry.

Breaking Down The Walls

In 2021, myself and a couple of other partners founded a non-profit organization called the Health Data Synthesis Institute (HDSI). Its goal is nothing less than to transform the world of scientific research into healthcare by encouraging and enabling collaboration. This is, I believe, a crucial endeavor in a world that is generating and measuring data at a prodigious rate.

The world needs this kind of initiative because there is still, unfortunately, an assumption that once somebody puts on a white lab coat, any desire for fame and fortune evaporates into the ether. The truth, as you're no doubt aware, is very different. Scientists are every bit as susceptible to the temptations of avarice and applause as any other discipline. With limited resources and funding, the scientific research community has developed a culture where individual scientists can become more focused on protecting their own project than on the wider goals of progress. This leads to a reluctance to share information and strong pressure to avoid challenging any existing axioms, to remove the risk of a quickly curtailed career.

As the CEO of HDSI, this is the culture I'm seeking to upend.

HDSI sets online challenges that address major global and local healthcare research topics and invites scientists to propose solutions. Submissions will be assessed by the Scientific Advisory Council and prizes will be awarded for the most innovative and workable ideas. Critically, ALL solutions developed and submitted for evaluation will, by default, be freely shared with the rest of the world so that any scientist can take a strong idea and develop it further.

In the short-term the hope is that this will lead to the development of new, powerful treatment protocols and therapeutics. In the long-term the mission is to change the culture of scientific research into healthcare so that the sharing of ideas and research data for the benefit of all becomes the norm rather than the exception.

Do not worry. Your mission is far simpler.

It Starts from The Top

The method that HDSI is using to change the culture of scientific research is a mixture of challenge and reward. These are just two of the tools at your disposal that will be explored in this chapter. But whichever culture-busting strategies you use, it's all going to start at the top.

That means you.

So, as always, we begin by looking inward. Because it's of little use to attempt to train your team into an era of better communication and accountability, if your own practice of communication is poor and if you're unwilling to take proper accountability for your own efforts.

It's not a case of leading by example – which is essential – but also being able to instill important cultural ideals that you truly believe in as evidenced by the way you look after your own work.

Just as we did in the opening chapter, with the subject of change, take a few moments to list all of the key qualities you want to see in your departments (communication, coordination, accountability, fiscal discipline, good record-keeping, etc.) that will enable you to make your high-performance CIO journey a success. Once you have that list, consider each element in turn in terms of your own abilities. Try rating yourself in each area out of five where…

5 = Exceptional

4 = Above Average

3 = Meets Requirements

2 = Below Average

1 = Needs Improvement

Next, talk to one or more trusted colleagues and ask them to rate you in each area. Compare the results and you may find some interesting gaps in your skills that need some work. If you consider yourself, or your colleague considers you to be, lacking in certain areas, there's no cause to be despondent or convince yourself that you need to put all of your plans on hold. It simply means that whatever strategies you put in place with your departments to improve those particular skills, need to count double for yourself.

Now Work Your Way Down…

You likely already have a fair idea of what the culture of your organization is, and where its strengths and weaknesses lie. But do not rely purely on your own understanding. Some formal assessment is crucial at this stage.

There are any number of ways in which you can review your teams – such as talking to team leaders – but I would encourage a more formal, systematic approach. The method I use is simple to understand, offers two levels of detail, and has the primary virtue of being an exercise you can repeat at intervals to monitor improvement (or lack thereof).

Create a simple chart that allows every person in the department to rate themselves out of five (using the same scale as earlier) on a variety of essential skills, while at the same time, allowing them to rate everybody else on their team using the same measure. Next, average out everyone's scores for each discipline so that, for each person, you can see how they've rated themselves compared with how the rest of the team views them.

Essentially this is a larger version of the exercise you've already carried out for yourself. It might look something like this:

	Personal Assessment	Team Assessment
BASIC SKILLS		
Listening	3	3.2
Communication (via email)	2	2.9
Communication (with peers)	2	2.8
Communication (with reports)	3	3.1
Communication (in small groups)	3	2.9
Communication (in large groups)	3	3.5
Facilitates effective meetings	4	3.1
Effective team leader	3	3.2
Manages work/life balance	4	2.5
Financial management	4	2.5
Strategic thinker	4	3.7
MANAGEMENT SKILLS		
Ability to manage employees	3	2.6
Courageous conversations	3	3.2
Manages difficult issues	3	2.9
Open, honest communication	3	3.3
Holds team accountable	2	3.2
Expectations management	2	2.7
Trusted by employees	3	2.6
Ability to accept and manage change	2	3.1
LEADERSHIP SKILLS		
Perceived as a leader	3	3.4
Discretionary effort	3	2.8
Models high performance	2	3.4
Respects / Leverage separate realities	2	2.7
Curious (but not judgmental)	3	3.1
Holds self-accountable	4	2.1
Acts as a change agent	2	3.6
Supportive of others' efforts	3	3.2

Figure 4.1 Sample Skills Assessment Framework.

The ultimate purpose of this exercise is because, as CIO, I am responsible for the growth of my team, and I need to make sure that I'm capitalizing on their strengths and tackling their weaknesses (if they exist). I want to help everyone become stronger and better in their role, yes, so that they can do a better job for our organization, but also so that they feel more confident and fulfilled in their role.

This data is obviously valuable to you because you can discover the mean of each skill across an entire department. But also take the time to go through the results with each person you ask to complete this exercise. The obvious places to start are where someone rates themselves significantly higher in a particular area than their colleagues. The goal is not to embarrass the individual, but to help their perceptions align with reality and feel motivated to do better. The conversation might go something like this…

"So, John, I want to draw your attention to the self-accountability category. You have rated yourself as a 4 out of 5 in this area, but the average score across your colleagues is 2.1. Why do you think this might be the case?"

"I don't know. Maybe the rest of the team doesn't understand the efforts I put into this area."

"That's possible, but it's unlikely that everyone has made the same mistake. Look at it this way, John. Why do you rate yourself highly in this area?"

"I know when I've made a mistake and I make a mental note to try to do better. It's something that's really important to me."

*"That's good. But what do you do externally
that lets your colleagues know that you've
acknowledged an error and that you've
taken practical steps to resolve it?"*

*"Erm... I don't know, I've not really
thought of it like that."*

*"That's okay. Remember, this is not about being
critical, it's about identifying ways in which we
can all improve. What do you think you might
be able to do to improve in this area in a way
that will be noticeable to the rest of the team."*

"I'm not sure, I'd need to give it some thought."

*"Sounds good. Think about it and if you
need some suggestions or if you think you'd
benefit from some additional training, just
let me know and we'll chat some more.
We're going to run this survey again in six
months so let's see what we can do to get
those two numbers more in alignment."*

In the reverse scenario, where their colleagues have rated them *higher* than their own personal assessment, it's also important to discuss with them why they think they might be underestimating their own abilities. There might be a confidence issue that can be addressed with an open conversation or some personalized training.

Most importantly, preface this entire exercise with a clear instruction that this is about establishing training needs and is not in any way a precursor to redundancies. It's critical that your team sees this as a positive exercise in which they're able to gain an understanding of their own strengths and weaknesses and be afforded opportunities to grow and improve.

Be prepared, however, for some negative responses and even some strong pushback. John, in the above example, has developed a negative reputation among his peers and he needs to address it. I would be following up with John over the next few weeks and months to see what steps he's taking to improve and to offer ongoing support. But if he's unwilling or unable to improve then I would likely need to have a courageous conversation about whether this is the right role for him or even the right organization.

Another occasional objection, when the team has rated someone considerably lower than their own perception, is that the rest of the team is wrong or is being malicious. It takes some real gall to make this kind of claim, but it's easily countered.

"So, John, I want to draw your attention to the self-accountability category. You've rated yourself as a 4 out of 5 in this area, but the average score across your colleagues is 2.1. Why do you think this might be the case?"

"It doesn't surprise me, to be honest. There are one or two people on this team who just don't like me and have obviously used this opportunity to make me look bad."

"Well, I'm sorry to hear that there is some conflict within the team, but keep in mind that this is an average across everybody. If it was just one

*or two people marking you down unfairly, then
the rest of the team would make up for that. This
figure indicates that this is the view of pretty
much everyone. So, perhaps we can focus on
how we can help you improve in this area."*

*"I don't have a problem in this area. I'm telling you,
the team just wants to push me out. It's obviously
not just one or two people, it's everyone."*

*"Well, that's really concerning, John. If the
whole team is unhappy with you, I'm forced
to wonder why that's the case. What has
been happening that has led to the entire
team being upset at you and what do you
think we can do to turn this around?"*

This is one of the real strengths of the process. Because the whole team is involved, it's very difficult for anyone to argue the results. What this hopefully allows you to do is turn the focus to how you can help the individual improve. I've had the odd situation where the entire team was upset at someone and they just refused to yield. I try to coach people in that situation and encourage them to take a humble view of themselves and be accountable, but sometimes people are just impossibly rigid. This exercise at least helps you identify when someone is a drain on the rest of the team, isn't coachable, and needs to be moved on.

Fortunately, those situations are rare. Most of the time, the ratings just show modest differences that help people identify where they're doing well and where they can improve. And that is good for all concerned.

Finally, aim to repeat this exercise quarterly or at least every six months. This gives you the ability to assess improvement in individual skills. Because here is the real diamond in this process…

As people improve their abilities in the kinds of areas listed above, this will have a positive impact on the culture of your department. And it works because it's not some nefarious or manipulative strategy but is instead a transparent process in which everyone is personally involved in their development and can see measurable improvements in themselves and their colleagues.

It'll take some time to get everyone to complete the survey so begin the process now and move on with the next steps below while you're waiting for the results to arrive.

Keep It In-House

I have no argument against the value of external consultants. I have been one myself for many years and I have on many occasions provided great benefit to my clients by providing such service. But sometimes you have a situation where a consultant has been with an organization for so long, sometimes years at a time, that they're virtually an employee in all but name. This is not desirable because, typically, consultants or freelancers cost a lot more than employees. That's a drain on your budget and, perhaps more importantly, the pay gap can create resentment among the rest of your team. This can even lead to disgruntled employees leaving, taking all their abilities and potential with them.

Far better to invest time and money in internal resources who are far more likely to stay with your organization long-term.

I urge you to assess exactly how much of your resources are being spent on external agents. In general, I use staff level consultants when I can't hire new people, when I need the resource for only a short term, or if it's a very specialized skill set.

Review the outside assets on which you rely and look for ways to scale it back. Not just so that you can free up funds for other, more important projects, but also so that you're motivated to develop more inhouse skills. One fully trained and developed employee, with a strong focused skill set, is more valuable to your organization than 2-3 consultants.

Along the same lines, look back through your calendar for the last 12 months and make a list of how many times you've had meetings with people, other than at board level. That includes meetings with your IT team, but also meetings with other departments at all levels, from upper management down to entry-level roles.

Yes, I know we'd all prefer to take part in fewer meetings but changing the culture of your organization as a whole cannot happen if you keep some people close, but others at arm's length. There are ways to improve your direct contact with a significant number of your employees without tying up excessive chunks of your time.

Create Your Culture Club

We've done some solid preparation, and now we're ready to begin the creation of your own high-performance culture. These are the actions I recommend you take during your first 90 days.

1. **Prepare people for change**

We have already touched on the importance of preparing yourself for change. Preparing everyone else is no less critical and is in many ways harder. Never forget that it is an unusual person who readily and happily embraces change, and that negative reactions are much more likely. Be prepared for defensive arguments, complaints, ultimatums, even tears.

Be gentle and empathetic, but do not yield. There is a fine

line between tolerance and permissiveness. Be prepared for the hard questions: Why me? Who made these decisions? What options do I have? Who else is impacted? What will I do now?

If emotions are running high and the tension is uncomfortable, don't hesitate to end the meeting and reschedule for a later time when the person has had more opportunity to digest the personal impact.

Appreciate also that resistance to change may not be visible on the surface. Just because someone smiles and nods at you doesn't mean they're onboard. You are part of the senior management team and what someone says to those in a position of authority like you may not align with how they really feel. It is the rare breed that can genuinely speak truth to power.

When you introduce someone to a new process, method or attitude, take the time to engage with the person and their feelings and concerns on the issues. Don't just monologue and assume that your charisma alone will get the job done. Encourage the person to express their feelings and be open about the fact that you don't have all the answers. Empower them to look for obstacles in your plans and encourage them to volunteer solutions or alternatives. Aim to end every meeting on a positive note.

Ultimately, getting people to accept change – even if they don't vigorously embrace it – is about selling your vision and convincing them that it's in their best interests to support the project. This means, plain and simple, helping them to see how this is going to benefit them in the long run. A more efficient department means, for instance, fewer fires to put out, less project congestion, less overtime, and so on.

Clearly identify the benefits of the change to each individual and you stand the best chance of keeping everyone onboard.

2. Instill leadership principles

If culture change is going to come from the top, it can't

emanate from you alone. Managers and team leaders at every level need to share your vision and your methods. It does no good if you're preaching one method and attitude and the leaders below you are contradicting you. When it comes to getting buy-in for your long-term project, getting managers on board is the golden ticket.

Create a charter of leadership principles that you want your managers to follow and create training if necessary. Your list may include the following…

+ Listen to what your team has to say and be engaged in every interaction.

+ Be yourself, be real at all times (don't have a management voice or persona).

+ Be caring and treat others the way that you would want to be treated (no matter if you meet them in the boardroom or the boiler room).

+ Lead by example in going above and beyond whenever and wherever possible.

+ Model higher performance by being diligent, ambitious and proactive.

+ Appreciate that everybody sees the world a little differently and learn to use the disparate perspectives at your disposal.

+ Curiosity is more powerful than judgment (be interested in your team and their feelings, but don't interrogate).

+ Be accountable and don't ask anyone to do anything you don't believe in and wouldn't be prepared to do yourself.

- ✦   Banish the "someone else's problem" mindset and address potential problems quickly.

- ✦   Provide clear and specific direction (never assume that you've been understood – follow-up and repeat instructions if necessary).

- ✦   Tailor your leadership approach to each individual's needs.

- ✦   Progress not perfection! (set realistic, progressive targets and celebrate every win).

3.   Champion engagement over communication

Memos and emails are fine for everyday communication. But if you want to change the culture you need to prioritize direct interaction with individuals. Group, face-to-face meetings are good. One-on-one meetings are better.

Make it your goal in the next 90 days to have as many one-on-one meetings with as many executives at your organization as possible so you can share with them your long-term plans, invite them to join you in the journey, and elicit their feedback.

Yes, this is a time-consuming undertaking, and it probably isn't an exercise you can repeat on too regular a basis, but this is critically important if you expect people to take your plans, and your determination to change the way things are done seriously.

Start with the highest levels of management and work your way down. Use the meeting to explain what you're working on, and what that person's specific role is going to be in helping you achieve a successful outcome. As you go down the list towards people with less responsibility, your instructions to them may become simpler, but find something for every person to take ownership of that will keep everyone moving in the same direction.

After you've completed your round of one-on-ones, set-up a monthly lunch meeting and invite a different group of people from your team, say around a dozen, to join you. Keep it casual and simply invite people to talk about what they're working on, what their obstacles are, and if they have any interesting ideas or initiatives they'd like to share.

Next, establish a quarterly team-wide call (phone or video call) that everyone can attend. This doesn't afford a lot of room for discourse, but it's an opportunity to update everyone on your progress and to commend people for their hard work.

Finally, create an annual event, where you get everyone together, in person, to build up a sense of team spirit and community. It's up to you how you organize this, but in the past my approach has been to rent a community college hall, get everyone under the same roof, and spend the morning updating everyone on what we've achieved in the last year. I would get each member of the leadership team to do a presentation. Afterwards, we'd have some lunch and then we'd all go bowling and have some fun. I'd literally rent out an entire bowling alley, group everyone into teams, and create some friendly competition, give out prizes, etc.

All of this is going to work towards helping people feel engaged in what you're trying to achieve. Your success is going to be their success and they should experience the benefits of what you're accomplishing. These practices are also going to increase your visibility, but most importantly your approachability. This is going to go a long way to developing a culture of progress that has real momentum.

4. Meet your vendors

Now we're really digging into some "next level" development. This step is the kind of thing that every CIO should carry out, but few take the time to do so. You're going to make a list of your top ten vendors, and then you're going to invite a senior representative from each to attend a meeting. You're going to get them all together in one room.

Start by explaining that you are creating a long-term initiative and that you want to adjust your relationship with them from "vendor" to "trusted partner." Then take them through the same presentation you've given to the board, your leadership team, and your executives. Map out of your long-term plan, what you're aiming to achieve, and how you intend to do it. Finally, invite each vendor to comment and offer suggestions as to how they can help you get where you want to be.

Spend a full morning with them. Pastries and coffee on the table. Make them feel special, but also make it clear that to be considered true business partners, you need them to reciprocate.

An example of how meeting with your vendors sets the tone going forward can be seen in how you handle contractual agreements. In Chapter Eight we'll be discussing how to take control of your budget by ensuring that contracts over a certain value have to be reviewed by you before they're signed. When I have the initial meeting with the top vendors, as part of my explanation of the new procedures I'm putting in place, I emphasize that, in the future, they need to ensure that I have signed off on any new contracts.

And if they try to bypass that, and a contract gets signed off without my approval, I might not pay it.

This has actually happened on more than one occasion, where a vendor accepted a signatory other than myself, and I was then able to go back to them and say, hey, remember when we discussed that unless I authorized the contract I wouldn't pay it? Looks like you want to test that theory.

The discipline you're going to put in place across your organization is only going to work if everyone is on board, external agencies included, and you're committed to enforcing the rules.

Ultimately, this meeting accomplishes three things:

First, it allows you to get a good understanding of which vendors are truly assets to your organization and which see you as little more than a number on a spreadsheet. This is going to help you down the line when it comes to better directing your IT budget.

Second, it allows you to identify the vendors who can genuinely help you make big leaps forward in your progress, especially when it involves changes or evolutions of the tech you use to improve patient outcomes.

Third, you've now let them know that they are your partners and they will be more likely to share in the pain when budget reductions become necessary or you're experiencing some serious technical difficulties.

If there is a feeling in your brain saying that this sounds a bit out of your comfort zone and maybe you can get by without it, push back hard. I cannot overstate how valuable this is to your long-term progress. What typically happens is that the vendors feel, and will express, genuine appreciation for being brought into your inner circle and for being identified as a key vendor. Most of their customers, even the ones with larger accounts than yours, will rarely if ever engage in this kind of exercise, so for the sake of a half-day meeting and some prep work (make sure you consult with your colleagues over which vendors to include), you can massively improve your relationship with your vendors and, as a result, your costs and your outcomes.

Oh, and those vendors that *do not* get invited, they're going to find out and they're going to feel it. That is not a bad thing. If they reach out to you to ask why they weren't included, be upfront and let them know that their service is simply not as valuable or productive as they might have been taking for granted. *"But, hey, while we're talking, what do you think we can do to improve that?"*

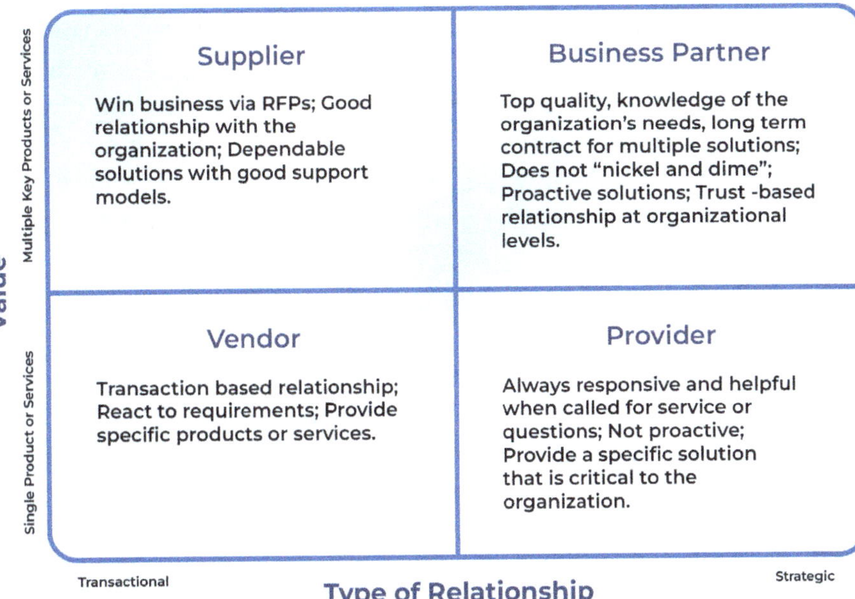

Figure 4.2 Vendor Relationship Matrix.

Having a culture of engagement is so valuable that you should be seeking to extend it to external organizations and vendors with whom you have a relationship. When you consult with your colleagues over which vendors make your top ten, focus on those who are already the closest to the top-right quadrant, and aim to get them all to that status.

5. Remove intransigent obstacles

Back to the Leadership Skills Assessment. Once everyone has completed their skills assessment, be on the lookout for team leaders who have a sharp gap between their personal assessment and the assessment of the rest of the team. In most cases, some training and coaching can solve the problem, but if the difference between the two is especially marked you should seriously consider taking permanent action.

Naturally, we never rush to terminate someone's employment, but if during the first 90 days you identify someone who is going to be a serious obstacle to your progress, everyone will likely be better served by your taking action now.

For example, one time I had a member of my team who was very smart and very effective at getting things done, but he led by intimidation. His team members feared him and were more interested in staying on his good side than taking ownership of problems or issues that needed to be dealt with, and risk getting on his bad side. Note this: If someone has a good side and a bad side, this is usually a major red flag.

Observing more closely I noted that he ran roughshod over his subordinates during meetings, and he didn't hesitate to publicly humiliate people if he disagreed with them. He was what you might describe as "hard-nosed," and I don't see that as being a particularly good characteristic of a leader.

Letting him go was not an easy decision. He'd been with the organization a long time and had moved up through the ranks because he was renowned for getting things done. But this, unfortunately, had the effect of reinforcing his bad behavior as if he was in his senior position because of those bad qualities rather than in spite of them. Everyone was shocked when I made the decision to terminate him, but they respected my decision and understood why I'd done it. And the correctness of my choice was driven home by the fact that many people clearly felt relieved not to be working with him any longer.

Another time I had a member of the leadership team who was very responsive and gentle with the highest levels of management, but very strict and aggressive with everyone below her. Another individual with both a good side and a bad side. She was very successful in her role because she could get things done, but at the same time she undermined the rest of the IT department to elevate herself in the eyes of the senior executives in the organization. Everyone below the most senior leadership knew exactly what she was like, but they feared her because of her close relationship with those above.

This behavior had been going on for years and previous CIOs had turned a blind eye. Fortunately, I noticed very early on in my tenure what was going on and it was a fairly easy decision to dismiss her. Oddly she seemed grateful when I told her I was letting her go. Perhaps she had made an uncomfortable bed for herself and was happy to be released from it. She was a talented individual and I sincerely hope she went on to do great things at another organization and was happier as a result.

The lesson in each case is that bad situations need to be dealt with decisively. This doesn't mean wildly swinging the axe and removing employees that are simply below average. But when someone is toxic to those around them, especially if they are in a leadership role, their negative influence can render an entire team ineffective. Give them the opportunity to change if that's possible, but if they're too rooted in their ways, like a tumor, it's better to excise them early for the sake of the whole.

We Have Different Realities

Sometimes intransigent obstacles exist outside of your organization, for example, with one of your vendors. It can feel like your hands are tied in this situation, especially if the alternatives are out of your price range or unsuitable for your needs. But it's still possible to be proactive in this scenario, it just requires you to activate your networking skills.

On one occasion we were working with a major electronic medical records (EMR) vendor who were experiencing all kinds of problems. They were an inpatient EMR that had merged with an outpatient EMR, and, from my perspective, it looked like they were struggling to marry the two. Their pitch was that they were going to offer the best of both worlds by having one supplier for both types of patient, but I guess it wasn't as straightforward as they made out, or at least not as straightforward as they'd hoped.

A couple of years went by, and nothing was happening in the way it was promised. Key milestones were being dropped, the promised integration wasn't happening, and more concerning was that there didn't seem to be any urgency to improve the situation. My complaints seemed to be falling on deaf ears. I spoke to the CEO and his team and aired my complaints and was given a great response about how much things were going to improve in the near future. But of course, nothing changed.

After I felt I had given them sufficient time to make substantial improvements, I took the step of doing some research and finding out who their top ten healthcare clients were in the country. I contacted the CIO at each, described my experience, asked if they were having the same problems, and of course they were.

I still felt that we had to give the vendor the chance to resolve the issues, but we needed to light a fire under them. I went back to the vendor again, explained that many of their top clients were experiencing the same dissatisfaction and frustration, and that we'd like to arrange a meeting at their offices and hash it out.

Naturally, they weren't keen, but I kept sending emails and pushing, and eventually they agreed. So, now I'm at their head office, with the CIOs of their ten biggest clients, meeting with the CEO and the leadership team. The CEO kicked things off with some big talk – to his credit (perhaps) he was a great salesman – and he talked about what they'd achieved and how amazing things were going and how they're going to be even better in the future. Eventually I cut him off and laid it all out. What he was describing and what we were experiencing were two different things. We were experiencing completely different realities.

Everyone else began chiming in with similar opinions and any agenda this vendor had to sweet talk their way out of trouble dissolved very quickly.

I'd love to say that this marked the moment when everything was turned around, but they couldn't get their act together and, today, none of the people in that room are clients of that particular vendor. But if I hadn't taken the step of proactively reaching out to the rest of the CIO community and validating our experience, we wouldn't have had the opportunity to get into a room with the vendor and confirm that, as we'd feared, things were never going to improve, and we had no choice but to find a replacement. We might have wasted several more years of time and money waiting for a working solution that was never going to appear.

This is one of the virtues of rejecting passivity. But keep in mind that, as with the above example, being proactive doesn't mean making knee jerk reactions. You should always be willing to give people time to change and come good on their promises. Just be willing to place limits on your patience.

6. Create rules of engagement

Create a pact with the leadership team, which will eventually filter down to the rest of the organization, to deal with disagreements or problems swiftly, in a professional manner, and most importantly in a way that maintains the cohesion of the team. Here are a few of the practices that I actively encourage:

+ Always give each other the benefit of the doubt when a problem arises and don't jump to conclusions.

+ If an issue needs resolving, don't send an email. Pick up the phone, talk about it, and establish the facts.

+ Look for separate realities and be prepared to discuss them, really making an effort to understand what the other person is saying.

+ If it seems like you're all spending too much time putting out fires, make a conscious effort to slow down, confront differences in opinions and methods, and reach a consensus on how to move forward.

+ Have each other's back at all times. Don't put up with any negative talk or gossip about someone who isn't in the room.

+ Do not hoard knowledge. Share it freely so everyone can be successful.

As always, these rules are only as effective as your willingness to enforce them. On one occasion, one of the deputy CIOs (I tend to refer to them as site directors) was breeding some irritation among the rest of the team. He was being critical of the IT team behind our backs and he was refusing to follow agreed processes. For instance, if a member of the medical team got locked out of the system and needed their password reset, there was a clear procedure that involved the person contacting the helpdesk so it could be dealt with systematically and the incident recorded. But instead of supporting that policy he would say "sure, I can help you," and just do it for them.

Maybe he thought he was being helpful (and that's a big maybe), but the reality was that he was undermining his team members by not being supportive of their efforts, and gave the appearance that he was trying to curry favor with other department heads.

This was reported to me by several members of the team, so I asked them to put their concerns in writing and that I would handle it. Once I had enough information for me to be confident that this was a genuine problem I brought the person into my office, sat him down, and told him that we were going to have a good, open, honest conversation because what he was doing wasn't right, his behavior was being observed by his colleagues, and it was hurting the unity of the department.

I didn't shout and scream – that isn't my style – but I made it very clear that this behavior was unacceptable and that he needed to tell me what he was going to do differently, going forward, to put it right, so that he could stay as a member of the team.

To his credit, he accepted the discipline, adjusted his behavior, and eventually became one of the strongest members of the team. Ultimately, I think this incident opened his eyes to the fact that people were observing his behavior and drawing conclusions. And that is a good truth to acknowledge. A culture of communication and trust only exists when everyone plays their part. As leaders people watch what we do and respond to that far more than anything we say.

Your new culture needs to be embraced by everyone, and those that cannot or will not play ball need to be moved on. But once everyone's pulling in the same direction, and contributing to that healthy culture of high performance, you'll start to see things falling into place.

To-Do List: Part Three
(Your 90-Day CIO Strategy Overview)

☐   **Task #1** – Write out a list of the skills and qualities that will be essential to creating your desired culture, and rate yourself on each. Ask other trusted colleagues to rate you and look for gaps in your abilities and attitudes that need improvement.

☐   **Task #2** – Expand this exercise across the rest of your teams so you can identify training needs. Meet with each individual and review their results.

☐   **Task #3** – Review the outside assets, such as consultants, that you're using and consider whether any of it can be scaled back, either now or in the future.

☐   **Task #4** – Look through your calendar and make a list of how many times you've had meetings with people other than at board level.

☐   **Task #5** – Create a charter of leadership principles that you want your managers to follow and, if necessary, build some training around them.

☐   **Task #6** – Arrange, within the next 90 days, to have one-on-one meetings with every executive at your organization to share with them your plans. Start with senior management and work your way down.

☐   **Task #7** – Set up a monthly lunch for around a dozen people in your team and invite a different group each month.

☐   **Task #8** – Schedule a quarterly team-wide call to update everyone on their progress and to commend their efforts.

☐ **Task #9** – Plan an annual event, involving every employee, which includes presentations from the leadership team, and some fun, team-building activities.

☐ **Task #10** – Meet your vendors and seek their assistance in meeting your long-term goals.

☐ **Task #11** – Identify any disruptive individuals among the leadership team and either coach them or let them go.

☐ **Task #12** – Create a pact with your leadership team to follow an agreed list of rules of engagement.

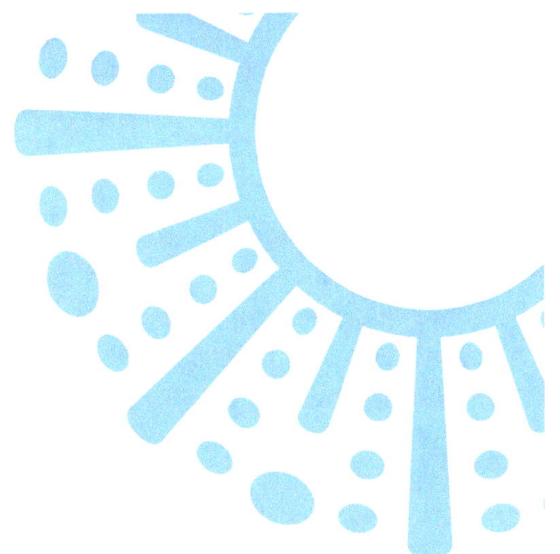

CHAPTER FIVE:

Engagement – Maintaining Core Focus on People, Teams, and Guiding Principles

During this past holiday season my son proposed to his girlfriend, and they agreed to commit to each other for the rest of their lives. They have come to know and love each other deeply during their relationship and they have a common vision of starting a family (hopefully more grandkids for us – hurrah!) and building their own happy ever after.

What a beautiful prospect this is. They are now officially committed to each other, but we refer to this stage of their relationship as: Engagement.

Planning out this chapter brought this to mind because although we tend to think of employee engagement in its simplest definition, that of being occupied or involved, I prefer to think of it on a deeper level. Not that employees should be engaged to their employer in some kind of romantic union, but engaged in the sense that there is a shared vision and commitment to accomplish something important and worthwhile.

To create a high-performance culture at your healthcare organization, you need everyone at all levels to be fully engaged with your plans and committed to seeing through the steps required to get there. This means they have to understand what you're trying to achieve, how you plan to achieve it, and what their important role is in making it happen not just for themselves, but for their colleagues and for the patients.

That's the type of engagement you must seek to instill in your team.

People, not robots

There's a lazy cliche, often seen in TV comedy, that people who work in IT are more comfortable with computers than people, and that unlike most of the world, they welcome the day when robots take over everyone's jobs.

I've no doubt that, like myself, you see technology as something that is designed to serve humans, and will never and should never be the other way around. But precisely because humans aren't machines, and have rich, inner lives, you can't create a simple program that will fully engage everyone in your plans.

The goal of this stage is to engage the members of your team so that they…

+ Are committed to the organization's mission, vision, and values.

+ Believe strongly that we can provide great care and outcomes for our patients and their families.

+ Understand the vision, mission, and values of the IT organization.

+ Are committed to the success of the entire team.

+ Are willing to go above and beyond the definition of their job (for example, would never say, "that's above my pay grade").

+ Come to work every day ready to give it their all.

+ Are active members of the team, not just participants.

+ Support each other regardless of the outcome.

+ Laugh and celebrate together.

There will be a small number of people on your team who instantly embrace all of the above, and an equally, or hopefully smaller number, who have no interest in developing any of the above attitudes. Those people, on both sides, are not your primary concern. It's the majority of the people in the middle who ARE capable of becoming fully engaged but need your help to get there that should occupy you.

Those people who sit in the middle are the worker bees. The people who are diligent, turn up on time, do their job, and leave promptly at the end of their shift. They're what we might call "good citizens" but they're not necessarily enthused by what they do and won't be easily excited by your ambitious plans.

In theological circles there's debate over whether it's better to be "righteous" or "good." Although being "righteous" sounds like the natural pinnacle for a religious person, it's actually the other way around. A "righteous" person does what is right in all circumstances but doesn't go any further than what they believe is reasonably expected of them. A "good" person, on the other hand, doesn't always get it right, but their intentions are genuine and, crucially, they're ready to go above and beyond the call of duty.

That neatly sums up what you're trying to achieve. You want your righteous employees to become GOOD employees. And that happens when they feel fully engaged in what they're doing, not just in the moment, but also in the long-term.

The temptation is to create a rigid funnel and force everyone through it, hoping they'll come out the other end in the shape you want them to be. But, it bears repeating, people are not robots and there is no inflexible strategy that will get the job done here. Instead, think back to some of the methods we covered in the previous chapter, in which we assess people (and get them to assess themselves) and then provide them with the training and mentoring they need to help them grow in their role, and potentially into a promotion.

Patience is key here. Apart from the aforementioned outliers who lack the humility required for growth and change (and who are unlikely to last in their role), everyone else WILL get to that fully engaged stage, but at different speeds and via different paths. Have patience and have faith in your people and you will get there.

Daily Service Review

Driving high levels of communication and engagement, and leading in this area by example, needs to be a constant endeavor. Everyone needs to know that we are being transparently honest with each other and that everyone is being kept in the loop. That's why the Daily Service Review call is so important.

Every morning, early, the leadership of my IT team gathers (either in person, or on a call) and check in with each other to find out what's happening in everyone's world. You can use a simple three question structure for the roll call:

1.) What have you accomplished since yesterday's call?

2.) What do you intend to accomplish today?

3.) What obstacles are you facing and what do you need to overcome them?

Simple questions, but the critical part is that everyone has to participate. No one can sit quietly in the background and just listen. This call, which some members may choose to attend in person, can be clunky initially, but once everyone gets used to it, you'll fly through it as everyone becomes accustomed to quickly summarizing what they've done, what they're doing, and what help they need.

This also helps to bring the team together. Often, when someone presents a hurdle they're facing, someone else on the team will chip in with a suggestion or an offer to help.

The idea is to get to 8am every day knowing everything that's going on in the IT department. You'll know what issues are brewing that might need higher level attention and what people are doing to support each other. And pleasingly, it's not just YOU that has this information. It is EVERYONE on your team. It's an incredibly powerful way to start the day that influences everyone's behavior and attitude.

Before long, your colleagues will also notice the difference because when they speak to you or a member of your team, at any point during the day – whether it's first thing in the morning or late in the afternoon – everybody knows what's happening and can intelligently explain the issues that are being addressed.

This level of communication and knowledge sharing among every member of your team only happens when genuine engagement is actively taking place.

The Daily Service Review is valuable, but no less golden are the other forms of communication we covered in the previous chapter. The one-to-ones, the weekly and monthly group communications, and the social events. But also, don't discount the benefits of casual communication that takes place when two team members run into each other in the halls or chit chat before and after meetings. Relationships form through these interactions and the working environment becomes more pleasant as a result. And when your team members are happy and engaged with one another, better outcomes result across the board.

We've all known a manager who, when they see two team members engaged in idle conversation, can't resist reminding them that there's work to be done. This doesn't make for a relaxed, pleasant working environment. The reality is that people's productivity is best judged by the outcomes of the projects they're working on, and whether they meet their targets and deadlines, not by whether they like to spend a few minutes sharing a video on their phone of their child taking their first steps.

When you truly respect and value your team, this kind of
latitude will come naturally. You can't, and most certainly shouldn't try
to, police how everyone spends every minute of their time. When you
genuinely appreciate how valuable your employees are and express that
appreciation, your people will believe that they're valuable as well, and
everybody gets a lift.

Again, this takes time, but it shouldn't take forever. There
will be, inevitably, a small but disruptive minority who don't have the
ability or the inclination to engage. It doesn't make them bad people; it
simply means they're ill-suited to working in a role where teamwork is
paramount. Identify these people early, make every effort to get them
to play ball, but don't be afraid to let them go if they refuse to make
any significant efforts. And make the call before they poison the well
and start to drag down other members of the team.

Additionally, I'm sure I don't need to advise you that this means
letting them go from your organization as a whole and not simply
moving them to a different department. Make the tough call and move
them on in the kindest and most humanistic way you know how. The
people on your team who matter the most will respect you for making
the right call and will appreciate the removal of a toxic presence from
their working environment.

People Before Profits

Don't worry, I'm not about to launch into a long anti-capitalist
discourse because I'm a strong believer that if there is no money there
is no mission. While optimal patient health outcomes is the priority,
that doesn't mean financial needs and challenges can be ignored. I am
also a strong believer that cutting staff should be an absolute last resort
and should never be done without exploring all other options.

I mentioned in an earlier chapter an example of a lack of
coherence between departments, as illustrated by the chief nursing
officer concerned about being short-staffed, while in the very next

meeting the CFO announced that we needed to cut five percent of the staff from every department, including nursing. I'm going to give you the specifics of the story (albeit with a few details changed so as not to embarrass anyone) because it's an excellent example of how to resist pressure to let go of valued team members. This not only keeps your department strong but also helps to create loyalty (another form of engagement) among your team as they recognize your willingness to go to bat for them.

In this example, the CNO was concerned about the number of infections occurring while patients were in our care and how that was affecting the readmission rate. His read on the situation was that we were short-staffed and the number of patients cared for by each nurse was too high. In the very next discussion, the CFO recommended that we cut the number of nurses to meet some previously stated financial goals.

There are two obvious ways to deal with this situation, and both are incorrect.

The first is to throw up your hands, say that it's out of your control, and make the requested reduction of staff. Effectively passing the responsibility, and therefore any negative consequences for the decision to someone else, namely the CFO and the financial team.

The second is to dig your heels in, refuse to even contemplate making the cuts, demand that the savings be made in other departments, and as a result create tension between you and other members of the leadership team who lead those other departments.

The third, less obvious but I believe to be the correct way to handle the matter is to argue that cutting staff from an already overworked team is going to cause more problems and will, in the long-run, only exacerbate any financial challenges that we are anticipating or are already experiencing. Offer instead to take it upon yourself to find the cost savings elsewhere.

In this instance, I spoke to the CFO and asked him specifically how much I needed to cut from my budget. The answer was $2 million, roughly the equivalent of 20 members of the staff. I told him to give me two weeks and I would come back to him with a plan to find the savings elsewhere in my budget. After that I updated him every other week on my progress so that, even though I didn't instantly find two million dollars in savings, he knew that I was moving the needle in the right direction. As a result, he stopped asking me to cut staff and instead we worked together to find a better solution.

Where in your budget can you find savings? I recently reviewed the IT budget for a healthcare system to familiarize myself with the organization. I specifically asked for the list of vendors and service providers to be sorted from high to low in terms annual spend. I quickly noticed that they were paying one vendor around a million dollars annually to "keep the system warm" years after it had been discontinued.

I had a similar experience with the same vendor at one of my other organizations. We were paying well over a half million dollars for them to provide access to the clinical data that had been stored in the systems many years earlier. This historical clinical data was clearly important, particularly if we needed to find archived patient information in the event of a lawsuit. But, after several years it was very rarely queried. As in, literally, you could count on the fingers of one hand how many times the data was accessed over a year, and yet we were paying all this money to store it.

Rather than complaining to the vendor and risking them locking everything down, I gave my team the project of downloading all the data and bringing it inhouse within the next three months. Once we were done, we cancelled the contract with the vendor (or, more accurately, we simply didn't renew) and saved that money from our budget. I'm sure that you can find the same if not similar saving opportunities if you scrutinize your budgets.

Not all budget savings are going to be on that level, but if you keep looking for opportunities to streamline or simplify, with the goal of reducing costs, you push back against the pressure to make personnel reductions when things get tough.

This is an indirect example of how leading your department with the right mindset, engaging with challenges directly, and prioritizing the needs of your employees and patients, can set the tone for a healthy, thriving team, all moving in tandem and engaged towards the goal of reaching that high performance state. But you must provide them with some guidance as they embark on this journey.

IT Guiding Principles

The meetings described in the previous chapter gives everyone a chance to give their viewpoints on your plans. If possible, you want to try and implement a little bit of everyone's input into the overall strategy so that everyone has a stake in what comes next. Everyone should be able to look at the written, laminated version of your guiding principles and see their fingerprints on it.

This is easier than it sounds because many of your executives will offer similar suggestions. Integrating the most useful and popular notions will dignify everyone with having played their part in what everyone is being asked to do.

You do, however, need to start with a framework rather than a blank piece of paper. You must create your own set of primary guiding principles, each with their own descriptors. You can tweak and add to this framework based on the input you receive, but you need to have something to show people that will drive the conversation, spark their imagination, and help them to understand what it is you're going to achieve.

This is another exercise in which the results will vary depending on your individual circumstances. But to help you get started, below is a more comprehensive set of IT Guiding Principles than those provided in Chapter 2. This is what I've used as a starter set in many of my organizations.

Commitment to Quality, Patient Safety, and Coordinated Care

+ We will put the patient first in all decisions.

+ We will create an information technology environment that will encourage our patients to choose our organization for their primary healthcare relationship.

+ Enable consistent, evidence-based standards of excellence across all venues of care.

+ Enable the provision of the most personalized and coordinated care across all venues of care.

+ Deliver all the information needed by providers and staff to make the care decisions.

+ Facilitate the engagement of patients actively and effectively in their care.

+ Whenever possible, staff will be given the opportunity to retrain in order to acquire the necessary skills and continue to add value and maintain employment.

Timely, Definitive, Inclusive Decision-Making

+ We will have clearly defined responsibilities and levels of authority for decision making.

+ We will make informed decisions with appropriate urgency and stay on track by not revisiting well-made decisions.

+ Our decisions will be based on what is best for the organization as a whole, not what is best for individual members, departments, or groups.

Collaborative and Creative Problem-Solving

- ✦ We will exhibit consistent leadership behaviors as we lead throughout the organization.

- ✦ We will foster open discussion about issues and areas of risk and be creative in determining solutions and mitigation strategies.

- ✦ We will have collaborative processes and engage patients, end-users, and executives from across the organization.

- ✦ We will focus on delivering sound, operational solutions rather than perfect solutions.

Frequent, Targeted, and Accurate Communications

- ✦ We will be focused in our communications to ensure that physicians, staff, and leadership are kept informed about impacts to their work and changes to the way we deliver and manage care.

- ✦ Our corporate and local facility leaders will serve as program champions – leadership commitment to the overall IT strategy and specific programs will be demonstrable and specific.

Integrated Systems and Standardized Processes

+ We will align on enterprise technology solutions to ensure maximum integration across the health system and extending out to the community.

+ We will enable the standardization of patient care wherever feasible across the system and reduce variability.

+ We will develop secured technology solutions to achieve full operational efficiency across the care-continuum.

+ We will measure the impact of our work with goals, metrics, trends, and provide an analytics platform to support population health management.

Well-Planned, Efficient Implementations

+ We will plan our work and hold ourselves accountable to aggressive but achievable milestones and performance metrics, including financials.

+ We will be creative in the development of learning materials to ensure efficient, scenario-based training and quick end-user adoption.

+ We are committed to strict quality assurance and adhering to defined testing, data migration, and change management processes.

+ The implementation of all solutions will be undertaken with a primary goal of enhancing our ability to function as an efficient system as well as reaching the financial goals established for the organization.

To-Do List: Part Four
(Your 90-Day CIO Strategy Overview)

☐   **Task #1** – Establish Daily Service Review calls/meetings to be completed no later than 8am each morning. Require everyone in your department to answer the following, or similar, questions.

       1.) What have you accomplished (since yesterday's call)?

       2.) What do you intend to accomplish today?

       3.) What obstacles are you facing and what do you need to overcome them?

☐   **Task #2** – Identify the individuals most resistant to engaging with these new initiatives. Seek to train and/or encourage them to participate, and if they're unable or unwilling, move them on swiftly, but humanely.

☐   **Task #3** – Acquire a list of vendors, ordered from high to low in terms of annual spend. Proactively look for opportunities to streamline, remove or bring the service inhouse.

☐   **Task #4** – Create your own set of IT Guiding Principles.

☐   **Task #5** – Share your IT Guiding Principles with your leadership team first and then with the other executives in the organization. Invite them to comment, tweak or add to your framework and content.

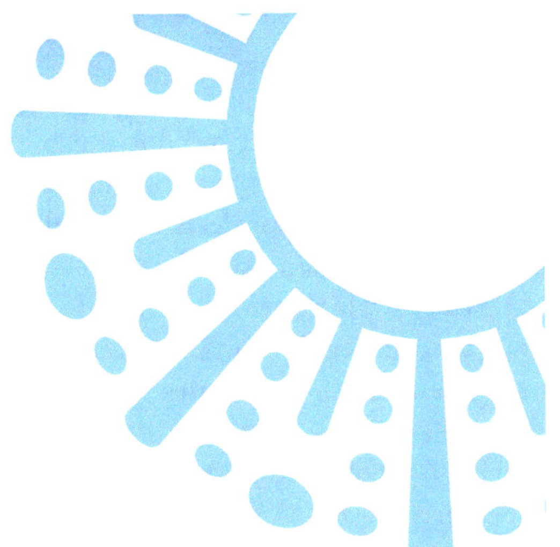

CHAPTER SIX

Accountability – The Entire Organization is Involved in Cybersecurity

There's a famous, darkly humorous webcomic in which a nerd imagines some criminals contemplating building a million-dollar hack to steal his cryptocurrency, only to be foiled by his 4096-bit encryption. In the next panel – the harsh reality – the crooks drug him and beat him with a $5 wrench until he coughs up the password.

This effectively illustrates the harsh truth that for every fiendishly complicated attack by hackers, there are many more simple acts of social engineering that aim to take advantage of people's misplaced trust and naivete. In fact, a 2021 study reported that 57% of attacks on organizations were social engineering attacks (tricking an individual into giving computer access, physical access, or data to an unauthorized person.)

Which is why this chapter on cybersecurity is primarily about accountability. Let's start with the fact that cybersecurity is a business problem and not a technology one. Nonetheless, a healthcare organization has to spend a lot of time and money on software and hardware that protects their systems from malicious attempts to break or breach them. But the biggest liability has been and always will be the people that work alongside you. People in all departments are the weakest link and we need to transform them into our strongest firewalls when it comes to cybersecurity.

Strange to think that of all the chapters in this book, it is this one, a discussion on cybersecurity, which will likely remain the most timeless. Social engineering is hardly new and predates even the most rudimentary form of technology. Pickpockets, for instance, for millennia have taken advantage of people's willingness to place valuable items within easy reach, making the ill-advised assumption that people will respect the ownership of their belongings.

Sad to say, but one of your most important projects in the next 90 days is to establish practices that train people to be suspicious of any email, text message, social media message or phone call that invites them to share sensitive information.

Everybody's Accountable...
But It Starts at The Top

At the time of writing, there was a news report about a Chicago-based health organization that has been hit with a class-action lawsuit over a ransomware attack. More than half a million patients saw their data breached and are accusing the organization of failing to follow basic security procedures. The financial exposure to this firm is colossal.

Needless to say – but I'll say it anyway – protecting your healthcare organization from cyberattacks is one of the most important functions of the modern CIO. The unvarnished truth is that if your company is the victim of a significant hack, you can expect to be shown the door within just 12 months. This is a critical area to address, and it's your own accountability that is going to set the tone. Because although every individual has a responsibility to act with due care, that doesn't mean anyone can be scapegoated.

If a frontline technician makes an error and exposes your organization to harm, they have to be accountable for that. But so does their manager for not adequately training them (or spotting their incompetence). And if their manager has failed in this area, then you've failed to give them the resources they need to teach and assess their team. In other words, every individual is accountable for their own actions, but every level of management is accountable for the performance of the people they manage. The level of accountability flows upwards, increasing through each layer of seniority, before landing finally on your desk.

Make this chain of accountability known because this is a crucial part of the culture of high performance that you're developing. When something goes awry it's important to be able to look in the mirror and honestly ask ourselves: "How did I contribute to this situation - for good or for bad?" When your colleagues see you doing this, they will emulate it.

I've worked with people who were quick to blame others when things went wrong, but equally quick to take credit when things went right. This kind of attitude destroys trust and crushes morale. You don't want those kinds of people working for you, and you certainly don't want to have this kind of reputation for yourself.

It's up to you whether you create a formal policy of accountability, but if you do it might look something like this:

1.) Open Communication: There are no foolish questions or ideas.

2.) Unconditional Support: Accidents and mistakes are learning opportunities and not excuses for punishment.

3.) One Team: As far as confidentiality permits, management will openly share information with their department.

4.) Training 365: Training in any essential skill will always be available on request.

5.) Transparency: Decisions at all levels will be clearly explained.

6.) Everyone's Responsible: Reject "someone else's problem" attitudes - report issues promptly.

7.) Create Your Own Solution: Never complain about a problem without having a suggestion for resolving it.

Review and Strengthen Your Security Systems

I recently had a lunch gathering with the members of a leadership team that I used to work with at a prior organization. Missing from the meeting, for no particular reason, was the Chief Information Security Officer (CISO) that I placed in his role. I was pleased to hear his colleagues agreeing what a fine job he had been doing in protecting their organization and that, to this day, they had never experienced a single breach.

All credit to my former colleague for this feat, but I think I can safely say that one of the reasons for his success is because I supported him in creating a culture where focus on cybersecurity was high and he was given the resources he needed to proactively protect the organization. This is a priority I've striven for in every CIO role I've held.

During the next 90 days there are a number of actions and programs you can put in place to strengthen your organization's cybersecurity. Start by reviewing the following areas:

- **Your Security Plan**

Review the written plan you have in place (if you don't have one already, drop everything and make this priority number one). It should clearly describe what resources and practices you have in place, and what projects are currently in development to strengthen the safeguards on your systems and data. Make sure it's fully up to date and then share it with department heads to make sure they understand what resources they have available, what is in development, and what they'd like to see improved. Finally, once you've updated this document, share it with the other members of the leadership team across the organization and make sure they're in full agreement with your goals and the financial investments you need to make it happen.

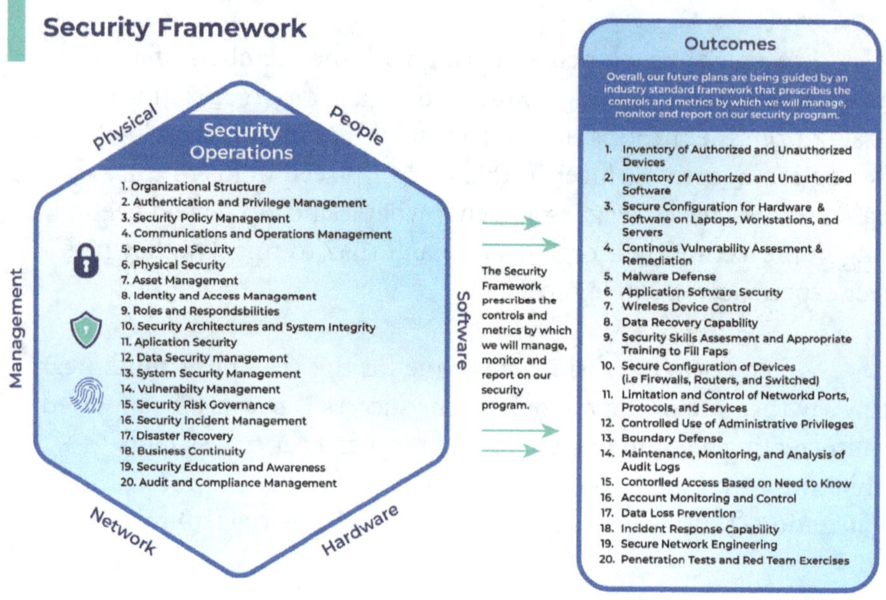

Figure 6.1. 20/20 Security Framework

As an example of what this might look like, one of the strategies I've put in place during my time consulting and as a CIO was a system I called the 20/20 Security Framework (see fig 1.) It's almost a cybersecurity strategy and plan on a single page. On the left-hand side are the 20 operations I'm responsible for – people, software, hardware, and so on – and inside that section are all the different activities that need to be carried out to ensure we have the right operating environment, from a cybersecurity standpoint, that will protect the organization as best as we know how.

On the right-hand side are the 20 outcomes that need to be regularly measured and assessed so we can see, at a glance, whether or not we're performing effectively or if there is more work to be done. I typically use a traffic light (green, yellow, red) system to rate each area and I create this report during the first month, when there are still a lot of improvements to be made. That way, everyone can see the improvements we're making over the coming months and can feel good about the progress being made.

In one of my CIO roles, we had next to no money to spend on cybersecurity. We basically had one guy looking after this area and as good as he was (he was ex-military and incredibly knowledgeable), it was too much work for one person. So, I convinced some members of the IT team that having extra knowledge in cybersecurity would be a great asset in their careers and would look great on their résumé. Effectively I got them to volunteer some of their work time to help out in this area on top of their regular duties and this gave us a good-sized cybersecurity team of nine people.

In practice, it's for the CISO to implement these items, but I am ultimately accountable for ensuring none of these areas are overlooked. I'm going to go into a little more detail on some of these areas in this chapter, but for a more comprehensive guide that will be valuable to your CISO, I can recommend the resources at fedramp.gov.

- **Plan Cyber Awareness Training**

It's not uncommon for new employees to be given a little training in this area when they first start their role – and already have a million other things swirling around their brain – and then the subject never comes up again. This is too important a topic not to repeat at regular intervals (perhaps annually), so if you don't have a regularly scheduled cyber awareness course, begin the process of creating one.

It might not be possible to create something from scratch within 90 days, but you can at least assign someone on your team to begin creating it, while also creating a schedule that will allow everyone in your organization to attend a session as soon as possible.

And I mean everyone.

That includes you and everybody from the CEO on down. Not just because they need it (no one is too "intelligent" not to fall prey to a cleverly crafted social engineering attack), but because it helps to establish that culture of accountability and confirms how important this training is.

If you want to speed things up and you have a budget, there's nothing to stop you from bringing in an external training company, at least for the first round of training.

The subjects to be covered in a cyber awareness training session are going to evolve over time as new hacking techniques are developed, but you should expect them to include at least the following:

Phishing: Fraudulent emails, text messages, voice calls, or social media messages that trick the recipient into handing over personal information, such as name, birth date, social security number, etc. Sometimes phishers cast a wide net, other times they target a specific person and create a phishing trap that uses something specific that they are more likely to fall for.

Pretexting: The fraudster pretends to be someone within your organization, usually at a senior level, and attempts to pressure the target into giving out sensitive information. Individuals who would usually never breach company policy by giving out sensitive data to a random person, can often be tricked into doing so if they believe they're being asked by upper management.

Baiting: An offer for something desirable, such as a gift card or set of tickets to a sporting or artistic event, in exchange for personal information. Email offers are common, but more sophisticated attacks could be, for instance, handing out free USB storage device gifts, which contain malware, at an event.

Tailgating: A criminal closely follows someone through a door so they can enter a secure location without an access card or pin number. This plays on social pressure not to appear rude by challenging people. It's amazing how often someone who is incredibly strict and, on the ball, when it comes to not giving out sensitive information over the phone or online, can fall for the trick of letting someone carrying a stack of heavy boxes through a secure entry without checking their credentials first.

A $60,000 Lesson

Email scams can be much more sophisticated than just exiled princes and unclaimed lottery wins. Sometimes a scammer will have done just enough prep to pull the wool over the eyes of people who would usually know better.

One occasion I recall was a mid-level financial manager receiving an email asking him to make an urgent $60,000 payment, and that it was critical it was sent by 11am. Under normal circumstances, this individual would have made a couple of calls to make sure it was legitimate, but there were two things working against him:

There was time pressure. The email made it appear that if the funds were not transferred immediately, something bad would happen.

The scammer had done enough research to find out the name and email of the CEO and made the email appear as if it came from this source.

It's hard to go to the CEO and ask if his request is real or a scam so he made a decision he likely still regrets to this day… he transferred the funds and then sat for half an hour and worried about whether he'd just made a massive blunder.

Eventually he did what he should have done in the first place – contacted the IT department and asked us to check the legitimacy of the email. It took seconds to figure out it was fraud (hovering the cursor over the CEO's name in the "Sender" field showed it was coming from an external email). We contacted the bank, but the money had already been transferred. We contacted the FBI, but there was little they could do. The scam was a success.

This is a good example of how a trusted member of staff failed to be an effective firewall that day. And it's also an excellent anecdote to share at cybersecurity training to illustrate how sophisticated scams can be and how important it is to double-check anything out of the ordinary. You'll likely have anecdotes of your own to share, but when you do, make it clear that challenging a request or completing a task late because you wanted to ensure that a fraud was not taking place will carry ZERO negative consequences. On the other hand, failing to carry out mandated checks on things like requests to transfer money, can result in disciplinary action.

- ## **Establish a Security Oversight Group**

Establish what I call a Security Oversight Group or SOG. You call it whatever you want but it needs to have leadership representation from legal, human resources, compliance, and finance. This group meets monthly to review the progress being made in the implementation of the security plans. More importantly, this group is the emergency response team in the event of a breach. They have a pre-established playbook that they will follow in such an event. The idea is that your planning will keep you and others from reacting to an event. Instead, you are executing a pre-determined plan.

Your SOG can also review any changes in the frequency or types of cyberattacks, which is why it's so important to track all events, no matter how small. For example, we always instructed our teams to be skeptical if an email didn't look right, but rather than deleting it to forward it to the IT team to review. This allows us to be proactive and, if an email is confirmed to be fraudulent, flush it out of everyone else's email inbox and block any further emails of this type. This kind of instruction to employees can be included in your cybersecurity training.

- ## **Check Your Cyber Insurance**

I would be amazed if you don't already have cyber insurance as part of your organization's existing security package, but don't assume that it's adequate for your current needs, especially if it hasn't been reviewed in some time. For example, you might have coverage against lawsuits and regulatory fines, should a breach occur, but you may also wish to have coverage for hardware repair and data retrieval. Naturally, insurance is not a replacement for solid cyber awareness training and penetration tests (more on this in a moment).

- ### **Hardware and Software Audit**

Reviewing your monitoring tools, firewalls, and countermeasures on a regular basis is critical. If this isn't part of your regular routine, make it so as soon as humanly possible. The goal should be to identify where weaknesses might exist, and which elements haven't been updated for some time.

Again, carrying out this process inhouse is preferable from a cost standpoint, but in the short-term there's nothing wrong with bringing in an external organization to audit your systems.

- ### **Create a Plan B**

No cybersecurity system is perfect, so do not make the mistake of assuming that because you've exercised due diligence in this area – maybe even going above and beyond – that you'll never have to deal with a breach or a serious, sustained attack. Work with your version of the SOG to decide now how you plan to respond to different scenarios. For example, if you fall victim to a ransomware attack, what is your policy going to be in terms of whether you pay the ransom or rely on backup systems to repair the damage? It's much easier to make a rational decision and come up with a sensible solution now than it is to react during a crisis – that's what I call SOG value.

Carry Out Regular Phishing and Penetration Tests

A few years ago, the University of Luxembourg carried out an experiment to understand what pressures might induce people to hand over a password. Randomly selected people on the street were asked for their attitude towards computer security. As part of the survey, they were asked to reveal a password.

Incredibly, almost one in three, complied.

The interviewers were strangers to the participants, but they were carrying bags with University of Luxembourg branding, so this created the impression that this was an official, and therefore trustworthy, survey. Even though, no doubt, it would be fairly easy for anyone to create bags containing the university's logo.

Here is the real kicker…

The participants were given chocolate as a gift for taking part. When the chocolate was handed over BEFORE they were asked for their password, rather than at the end of the survey, almost 50% complied.

It's possible the participants were just really, really into chocolate. But a more likely explanation is that, like most people, they were responding to the social pressure to return one favor for another. The power of reciprocation.

I'd be willing to bet, if you'd interviewed the participants before this test, and simply asked them whether they would give their password to a stranger, all of them would have said "no." And yet, in the right circumstances (or perhaps we should say, the wrong circumstances), almost half of them complied.

So, when you train your employees not to hand over sensitive information under any circumstances, and they readily respond, do not think for a moment that this means they're bulletproof. Far from it. This is why you need to carry out phishing exercises at least once per quarter.

For example, one of the tests I carried out previously was to create a nice-looking email in which the recipients were told they'd won free tickets to a New York Giants football game. If they clicked on the link, it would direct them to a form they had to complete with their personal information in order to receive these non-existent tickets. We sent this email to everyone in our organization, and anyone who was taken in by the email was given a warning.

And we took this seriously. Employees should not be opening these kinds of emails at work anyway, but if they do and they fall for this kind of phishing scam they are potentially a weak link.

Everyone who failed the test was told that they would be tested again in the future, and if they failed a second time, they would be suspended from work for two weeks without pay. If they failed a third time, they would be gone. How seriously do you think people took cyber security after they failed this test even once? I made this message loud and clear to the entire IT staff because, to my amazement, we were the worst offenders in the entire organization.

Some people will take the training, they'll get it, and they won't fall for this kind of scam. But some people won't connect the dots until they personally fail this test and realize how easy it is to fall down. And, of course, how important it is for them to take personal accountability for protecting sensitive information.

Put some time and effort into this exercise. Make sure the email looks good and looks legitimate because the real scammers, some of them at least, are creating very sophisticated, very realistic-looking frauds.

If you want to put a positive spin on it, look for ways to reward people for successfully avoiding or spotting a scam. You could, for instance, give a prize to every team or department where 100% of the members avoided the scam.

This isn't about trying to catch people out. You want them to succeed. But at the same time, you need to impress on people that they have personal responsibility in this area. And do not forget to move that accountability up the chain. If someone fails this test three times and is let go, their manager should also be put on notice because it means they haven't done enough to train their team.

If all of this sounds a bit strong, you haven't been paying attention. The financial and reputational costs to your organization if a real breach occurs is huge. Personally, you could lose your job if you're found to have been negligent. And most seriously of all, lives are at stake. If your patients miss appointments, get the wrong medication, or have to have surgeries delayed because of chaos stemming from a cyber-attack, this represents a serious threat to the wellbeing of the people you care for.

So, run these phishing exercises regularly, at least 2-3 times a year. Also, hire an external agency to periodically attempt to break into your network. This will expose any weaknesses that need shoring up. Most importantly, conduct annual training and awareness sessions for everybody. Take them seriously, and if you maintain that attitude, it will only be a matter of time before everyone else takes them seriously as well.

Remember that cybersecurity is job one for you and needs to be a major priority during your first 90 days.

Piggyback Training

Getting people enthused about another round of training, on top of all the existing mandated education and meetings, is never easy. So, if your organization already has a packed schedule, try piggybacking your cybersecurity training onto an existing set of regular training. If, for instance, there is an existing, mandatory, quarterly staff meeting, speak to the trainer and ask if you can have 10-15 minutes at the end (or the beginning) to run through some cybersecurity tips.

Alternatively, if your organization has a learning management system that new employees are required to review, and that existing employees have to use as a refresher at regular intervals, consider adding your training into the system so that it becomes part of the regularly consumed training content. This is especially valuable if it allows you to reach new starters early because they may be especially vulnerable if they're arriving from a different sector that doesn't see as many cyberattacks as healthcare.

Finally, if your organization is especially large, it may be more practical, rather than running in-person training, to create a short instructional video that teaches the basics of cybersecurity and explains how everyone can play their part in protecting the institution. As with the above suggestion, this can be shown at existing regularly scheduled meetings. Or it can be sent to every employee via email and the response tracked so you can see who hasn't gotten around to watching the video and who might need a nudge to make time for it.

To-Do List: Part Five
(Your 90-Day CIO Strategy Overview)

- ☐ **Task #1** – Review (or create) your security plan. Share it and obtain feedback from your department heads and make sure it covers the resources and policies you have in place, as well as the projects in development. Share the results with the CEO and the members of the cabinet and make sure that they support all of your ongoing and planned initiatives.

- ☐ **Task #2** – Establish your Security Oversight Group and begin the monthly meetings.

- ☐ **Task #3** – Plan and schedule regular cyber awareness training. Make sure every member of staff, regardless of seniority, attends.

- ☐ **Task #4** – Check what your cyber insurance policy covers and consider whether it is adequate for your needs.

- ☐ **Task #5** – Audit your hard and software cybercrime defenses and identify areas of weakness or that haven't been upgraded for some time.

- ☐ **Task #6** – Create plans that outline how you will respond to any future security breaches.

- ☐ **Task #7** – Carry out regular testing, such as sending phishing emails to everyone in the organization. Any individual who fails the test should be given a warning and advised that a second failure will result in a two-week suspension, and a third failure will result in termination.

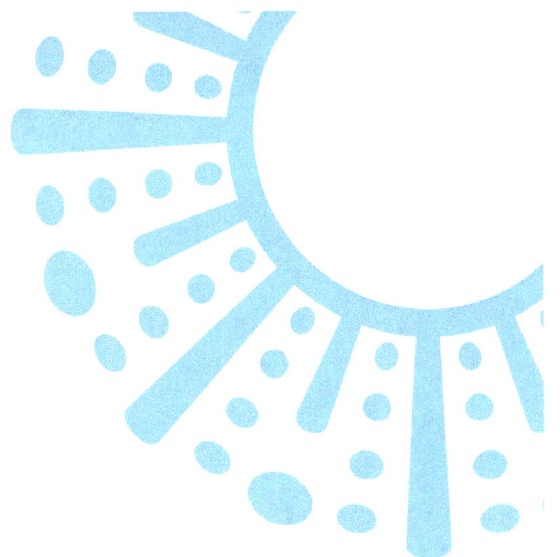

CHAPTER SEVEN

Operational Excellence – Driving Organizational Maturity

As we have discussed, you need to act like a general manager and an information technology executive at the same time. When asked by members of your family and friends what is it that you do, you need to be able to confidently say that you are part of the senior management team of your organization and have proven your ability to lead by example and thrive in the fast-pace, patient focused and operational-driven environment of today's healthcare. You've been a major contributor to reaching your organization's mission and vision in a distinctive, positive, and meaningful way. But you can't say that with confidence if your IT organization is not delivering the services expected on a day-to-day basis. That's the bread and butter of our job… the basics of what's expected of us. So, let's not get too far ahead of ourselves by thinking about high performance without first focusing on operational excellence. I have yet to see an organization that can go from the reactive stage directly to high performance. Before reaching the zenith, let's make sure that we're delivering excellent services and results that are noticeable at all levels of the organization.

Earlier I mentioned that there are three possible states for a healthcare organization (and to a certain extent, this can be applied to any organization):

1.) Reactive

2.) Operational Excellence

3.) High Performance

Now is a good time to look at the work you've completed so far, during your 90-day journey, and assess where you feel you are at this point. I provided part of this list in Chapter 2 but here is a more expansive list of defining characteristics of each stage.

REACTIVE STAGE OF ORGANIZATIONAL DEVELOPMENT

- Federated with operational silos.

- Disparate processes and technologies.

- Inconsistent communication and coordination practices.

- Immature operational tool sets.

- Focus on delivering short term results with limited planning.

- Perception by end-users lower than expected.

- Need for additional oversight and management of investments.

- Limited performance management and avoidance of courageous conversations.

- Low employee engagement scores.

OPERATIONAL EXCELLENCE STAGE OF ORGANIZATIONAL DEVELOPMENT

+ Plans clearly defined based on a consistent IT operating model.

+ Common processes based on standards.

+ Common deployment of mature tools set.

+ Constant communication and coordination with the elimination of silos.

+ Consistently applied effective business and IT practices.

+ High staff morale with higher-than-average engagement scores.

+ Best practices firmly imbedded in daily operation.

+ Meeting operational and financial metrics

+ Knowledge management functions fully implemented.

+ A model of transformational leadership.

HIGH PERFORMANCE STAGE OF ORGANIZATIONAL DEVELOPMENT

+ Value creation as the primary driver.

+ Anticipating business needs of the member organizations.

+ High level of end-user's satisfaction.

+ Highly supportive of coordinated care across the system.

+ Clinical systems that support the delivery of high quality, standardized care, based on evidence-based medicine.

+ Well above average engagement scores for all staff members.

+ A true learning organization.

+ Industry model for excellence.

Unless you began your journey from an exceptionally healthy state, it's unreasonable to expect that you've already reached the high-performance stage. Typically, this stage is only reached after several years of applying the practices, principles and strategies described in this book.

Equally, don't be alarmed if you see evidence that indicates you're still in the reactive stage. Many organizations exist permanently in this state and the fact that you're taking steps to move beyond this immature stage puts you ahead.

Ideally, however, if you're putting into practice what we've discussed in the earlier chapters, you should be able to observe some green shoots that indicate operational excellence is at least on the horizon.

Evidence-Based IT

The practice of evidence-based medicine is the foundation of modern medicine. The scientific process of research, and the approval process for medications and therapeutics as applied by the Food and Drugs Administration are all based on collecting convincing evidence that the intervention is going to be more beneficial than harmful to patients.

As progressive IT leaders we need to operate under exactly the same principle.

Today, most IT organizations follow some sort of discipline when it comes to programming, maintaining the technical environment, and supporting applications. But unfortunately, in my observations, the operational processes and disciplines are not enough. The level of consistency and discipline is just not there; certainly not to the level where it could be considered an operational excellent environment.

The idea of an evidence-based IT policy may sound strange, but I know from my own experiences that this is the preeminent method for turning an IT department into a high-performing organization.

The key to achieving this level of performance is the correct application of the Information Technology Infrastructure Library (ITIL).

ITIL: Best Practices

ITIL is a body of work that has been developed over decades to guide us in practicing what I consider to be evidence-based IT and this is the best method for getting you, first to the operational excellence stage, and eventually to the high performance stage. Just as with the clinical side of medicine, the ITIL processes provide a prescriptive set of guidelines for how we run all aspects of our operations. From how we interact with our end-users to how we maintain our server farms.

If you develop the culture of excellence we've already discussed and implement these disciplines as prescribed, the speed at which your organization matures is going to accelerate rapidly.

Although this is certainly not an ITIL manual or reference book (there are already many that have been published), it's important to understand the general concepts and components that are critical to implement in an operationally excellent environment. These assets are proven, industrial-strength business performance and service management tools, and should be the backbone of your development. If you embrace ITIL you can expect the following benefits:

+ Your IT services will be fully aligned with the requirements of the business (rather than merely reacting to changes and progress).

+ Your IT department will have a set of best practices that will guide their activity, while still allowing flexibility to develop creative solutions that fit specific conditions.

+ An optimal level of service provision at a justifiable cost.

+ A non-proprietary, vendor-neutral, technology-agnostic set of best practices.

Since it is outside the scope of this book, I am not going to break down every element of ITIL, but I am going to offer some recommendations based on the two modules that I consider the most important for your development: The Performance Management Suite and the Service Management Suite.

Performance Management Suite

What is not defined cannot be controlled. What is not controlled cannot be measured. What is not measured cannot be improved. Which is why Performance Management should be the cornerstone of any organization that believes in a culture of accountability. Metrics should be agreed with the business leadership and should be used to assess performance, and then to drive specific developments or changes.

The work you've done so far during your 90-day journey should be enough to create realistic metrics based on where your organization is today, but those metrics should change at various intervals to reflect your improvements. Metrics that are too easily achieved will not push your teams to progress and continuously improve.

Your metrics should include Service Level Agreements (SLAs) to measure service delivery and a management scorecard to record results and allow improvements, or lack thereof, to be observed.

Service Management Suite

Governance and financial discipline are the subjects of the next two chapters, so we won't dig too deeply into those topics now. Suffice to say that service management cannot be properly organized without getting your arms around these two areas. For now, note these four key processes, and we'll cover them in more detail in the next two chapters.

✦ Demand and Supply Management: For macro planning,

and balancing demand with funding and resource capacity.

+ Service Request Management: Enabling best practices for request and change management, while also eliminating non-value-added requests and their subsequent costs.

+ Time Management: An accurate accounting of where resources are being spent. This is going to be key for reaching the goal of allocating 80% of our resources to value-add activities and 20% to maintaining the environment (Pareto Principle discussed earlier).

+ Program and Project Management: Enabling the implementation of high performance strategies for delivering genuinely useful application functionality. This is critical for meeting the demands, including on-time and on-budget delivery of clinical, operational, and administrative solutions.

Request Management

It's not unusual for CIOs, if they take the time to sit down and make a list of all the current projects, large and small, in development, to discover they're attempting to oversee in excess of 100 programs. This is way too much to be able to produce results in any reasonable amount of time without scattering everyone's focus. Whittling this down to the 15-20 most valuable and/or critical projects as selected by the organization's leadership is going to help you speed up your progress and also help you keep a better grasp on your budget.

One of the keys to achieving this goal is the development of a comprehensive service request process that requires all prospective projects to be properly assessed before approval. This method will be covered in more detail in the following chapter.

Demand Management

This area refers to the collaborative process of working with the business to focus IT activities on areas that generate optimal value for your patients and their families, but also the organization as a whole. Naturally, not every piece of work you oversee will have the same level of priority, so this process needs a clearly defined set of rules so that decision-making and prioritization can be carried out quickly and efficiently. Key components of this process include…

+ A set of business rules that ensures IT capacity is prioritized based on the highest value activities, and that work can be completed in a cost-effective manner.

+ Adjusting the size of the IT organization based on available funds and agreed service levels. This also extends to filling under-utilized capacity with missing skill sets.

+ Maintaining a pool of resources dedicated to handle short-term needs (quick fix items.)

+ Establishing clear linkages between the organization units that are driving IT activities and costs.

+ An annual "work plan" updated quarterly, that identifies and schedules major initiatives and reflects ongoing break/fix and enhancement activities. The "work plan" should be arranged so that requested work will be delivered as cost effectively as possible.

+ A detailed staffing plan that balances supply and demand, and allows work to be completed within the defined timetable, scope, and cost. It also helps in identifying skills gaps that need to be address by training of the current staff, hiring for specific skills or reaching out to consultants on a short-term basis.

✦ Service levels that define severity-based response times and resolutions for each major request.

✦ Detailed tracking of performance against defined project plans.

✦ Continuous improvement driven by root cause analysis, corrective maintenance, and preventive maintenance activities.

✦ Well-defined request and problem tracking processes, supported by the effective use of tools.

Change Management

This process is responsible for controlling and managing requests related to changes in infrastructure, applications, or services. The goal is to effect these changes in a way that promotes the benefit to the business while also minimizing the risk of disruption to existing services. This area also manages the implementation of approved changes.

Organizational Alignment

This area is about having the right teams, of the right size, and with the right mix of skills to provide the most cost-effective services. When managed appropriately, this will allow you to keep costs down, while still offering adequate opportunities for individual career growth among your team members.

Consolidated Service Desk

Because of the acquisition nature of how healthcare systems have been put together, it's common to have different service desks for different parts of the organization. But operational excellence is virtually impossible without consolidating all of your service provisions into a single point of contact. This is not only cost efficient, but also resource efficient, with the added bonus that end-users will appreciate getting the support they need quickly and without being passed around from person to person until they find someone who can help them.

In this day and age, you should also be aiming for 24/7 service availability, 365 days a year.

Again, this is just a high-level overview of ITIL. Your service management team needs to absolutely understand all the details of the ITIL processes and establish an implementation plan. This is not a quick fix for your current operational ills. A typical implementation plan is approximately 24 to 36 months with visible, continuous improvements within the first nine months. Depending on your starting point, results may be achieved faster or slower in your organization. And remember, these processes will not only impact your service management team but your entire organization. It's critical that everyone is well aware of the implementation plan and educated on how their jobs will be impacted. This is part of that communications and engagement culture that I emphasized earlier.

If you have not already done so, I would encourage you to begin the development of your service management plan within the first 30 days, including the education and awareness sessions for the entire staff. This is a major step forward in your high-performance journey.

Minimizing Outages

When I am getting people at a healthcare organization on board with the concept of evidence-based IT, as I mentioned earlier, the simplest analogy is evidence-based medicine. This mode of treatment has been the standard around the world for some time and people already appreciate the value of only performing procedures when you know precisely what the expected outcome is.

The principle of evidence-based IT is the same. ITIL gives you a set of standardized processes that are proven to work if you apply them in the right circumstances. Which means, if you gather enough data and correctly analyze the situation, your solution will be the best one for the problem at hand.

For example, consider one of the key ITIL processes: Change Management.

Imagine, for a moment, that you discover a server problem, and you need to create a patch to resolve it. You know what the problem is, it appears to be a simple resolution, so you go ahead on your own initiative and make the change. Half an hour later three other servers and their applications go down. It's fairly obvious that the problem is due to a small error in the patch you uploaded, but you're on your lunch break right now and no one else in the department knows what you did.

By the time you get back to your desk, the whole team has dropped everything and is digging into the servers and applications to try to locate the problem. More applications have had to be taken offline in the process and some clinical departments, as a result, are at a standstill or have switched to manual processing which is highly ineffective.

Now you get the team up to speed with the root cause of the problem, but by this point, more patches have already been applied to the other servers to try to fix the problems caused by the original patch, and backing out everything takes hours.

This is what happens in a department where change control discipline doesn't exist (or it exists but isn't enforced with any consequences).

By contrast, if the department is running at an operational excellence level and ITIL processes are being followed, when you find the server problem, you report it to the change control group, and they approve the patch to be created and uploaded on an emergency basis the following day. At 7:15 a.m. the following morning, at the Daily Service Review, everyone is advised of the changes that are going to be made, including the patch you've created. Because everyone on the team knows what is going on and what updates are being made today, they know to look out for any potential problems.

The patch is uploaded at 8am and, unfortunately, it still contains a small error. However, because ITIL processes are followed, when the outage is reported, it's immediately clear to everyone where the root cause is and the servers are quickly rolled back to their earlier state while the patch is reviewed to locate the problem.

Instead of an outage that lasts for hours, you have an outage that lasts for just 15 minutes. And instead of a whole team having to take their attention away from their ongoing projects to fix the problem, the issue is resolved quickly and efficiently, requiring the attention of only one or two people.

What's interesting about this example is that the sometimes unavoidable human error is the same in both scenarios, but the difference in the levels of damage that resulted are tremendously different. That's the power of an engaged, well-disciplined team, that's uniformly using the ITIL processes.

To-Do List: Part Six
(Your 90-Day CIO Strategy Overview)

☐   **Task #1** – Assess your current processes and map them to ITIL.

☐   **Task #2** – Review your service management tools suite and make sure it supports the plan. If not, include procurement and implementation of new tools into your plan.

☐   **Task #3** – Develop an ITIL primer for the education and awareness of the entire IT staff.

☐   **Task #4** – Communicate your plan to the leadership team of the organization.

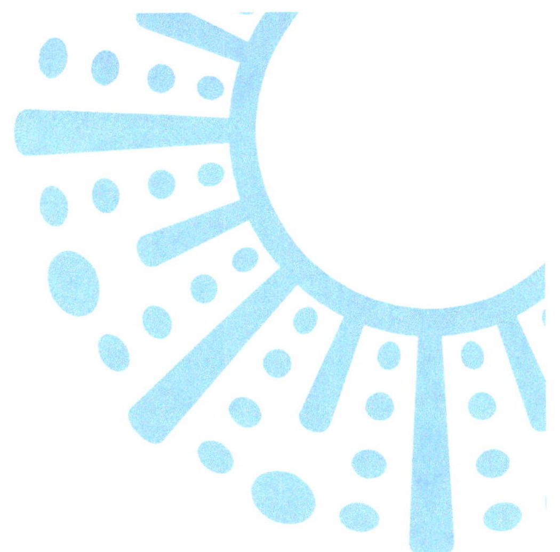

Financial Discipline – Minimizing IT Risk While Maximizing Innovation

You don't need to have been raised poor to have financial discipline, but it develops an attitude toward money that you can't get any other way. I'm sure this has helped me figure out a simple, but structured way of looking after my budget and ensuring the money goes exactly where I want it to go, and nowhere else.

As mentioned earlier, I was raised in a small town in the Dominican Republic along with my 12 siblings (seven girls and six boys, including myself). In the mornings we went to school, a small one-room building, and in the afternoons I helped my father sell the furniture that he made. We'd sell to people directly because this had the highest profit margin, and what we couldn't move we'd sell to a local store. If things went well, we'd get a penny to buy bread that was made fresh that day, instead of the prior day's leftovers which were hard and difficult to chew.

On the weekend, I'd go to the local baseball stadium and a guy there would give us little packets of roasted peanuts to sell to the people going in. After that we'd entertain ourselves by trying to jump the wall without being caught by the security guard so we could watch the game (the good old days growing up back in the Dominican Republic!).

So, yes, money was tight, but even then, I knew how to make what I had last. I saved as much as I could and would even sometimes loan money to other kids with interest. I was a miniature bank of one even as a kid.

I also found creative ways to make things stretch further. For instance, if we wanted to go to the movies, they wouldn't let us in unless we were wearing shoes, and most of us kids didn't have that luxury. So, we would get one pair of shoes among us, one of us would get into the cinema wearing them, and then throw the shoes out of a window for the next person to go in. In a short time, we were all watching the movie shoeless.

I don't miss the days of living so frugally, but I appreciate the financial discipline it instilled in me. There are always ways to make income and expenditure balance a little better if you have the work ethic and the smarts to make it happen. Even as an adult, this attitude has stayed with me. I used to own a series of beach properties that I would rent out. On a weekend, you'd find me sweeping and dusting, getting them ready for the next customers because the margins were better if I didn't have to pay for a cleaning company.

I taught my kids the same principles. If you have a dollar, live like you have 50 cents. Or, if you want to splurge, live like you have 75 cents. What you must never do is have a dollar and live like you have $1.25. You sleep infinitely better when you have full control of your finances, and you don't owe money to anyone.

Repeat: No Money, No Mission

IT budgets have become a major part of the overall finances of healthcare systems throughout the country. The increased cost of personnel, hardware, software, and services have driven the cost of IT dramatically higher in the last twenty years. Add to that the additional costs that we have incurred to keep cybercriminals away from our organizations.

In some cases, despite all of our advances, IT still has not been seen as strategic and, therefore, these expenses are seen as a necessary evil. Some organizations would rather allocate this money to build new facilities or expand clinical programs. Fortunately, this is becoming the exception rather than the norm as CEOs and other leaders have realized that without IT they cannot operate the organization or provide proper patient care. Not only that, but it's also clear there is no innovation without IT. As IT leaders, we need to continue to push this agenda until SOME becomes NONE. All healthcare organizations need to recognize the tremendous value of IT.

Here is a good example of that value recognition. In one of my organizations, we owned and fully operated a laboratory company. The President of that organization, who served with me on the system CEO Council, always described his organization as an IT company that processed laboratory specimens. He clearly understood that without IT he had no business because not only could he not process the specimens, but he also had no way of communicating the results with the ordering physicians or the patients.

I don't want to even insinuate that hospitals will someday describe themselves as IT organizations that care for patients, but they do need to realize that delivering optimal patient care is highly dependent on the availability of the solutions that we provide. That increased dependance on IT doesn't lessen our duty and responsibilities to be good stewards of the funds that are allocated to us. We need to maximize the value that we return to the organization for their investment in us.

I've also come to expect that my IT operating budget will not increase from year to year (unless we acquire other organizations during the year). As such, I know that I need to get more productivity from each member of the team in order to provide the expected value. Remember the discussion in an earlier chapter about the Pareto Principle and the need to go from 80% of our resources being applied to maintaining the current environment to 20% in the future? To get there we need to work smarter, apply the disciplines in our operating model, and drastically increase the productivity of each individual. This is why I usually increase the training and travel portion of my budget. An added benefit is that this is a clear sign to our team that we are committed to them and will continue to invest in their future. That's a powerful message that goes a long way in driving their engagement and commitment to the organization and the patients.

But, increasing travel and training budgets is a tall order since I don't expect or plan for any budget increases on an annual basis. If anything, my expectation is that the IT budget will increase by the rate of inflation which means that, in real dollars, we don't really have an increase.

By the way, I'm not referring here to the capital budget. With the governance model that we'll discuss in the next chapter, the capital budget by and large is determined by the projects that the organization approves. Of course, we manage that too but it's not allocated based on our needs but on the needs of the organization. This will become clearer when we discuss our intake process.

Back to the operating budget and how we can best manage it. Here is what I typically find when I arrive at an organization either as a CIO or as a consultant:

- ✦ No written policy about contracting and financial management in the IT department.

- ✦ Managers and above are all able to sign contracts that commit us to future payments.

- ✦ No dedicated staff for IT finance and contract management.

- ✦ Vendor contracts have built-in significant automatic annual increases that are not tied to the official inflation rate.

- ✦ Automatic payment to vendors for products and services that we have discontinued or no longer need (sometimes these contracts were entered into by a department outside of IT but we still carry it in our budget).

Taking Control

If you currently have an environment like the one above, what now? Here are the steps I take to gain better control of the situation:

- Set up a small department within IT that's focused on contracts and financial management. The leader of this team provides me with budget reports every two weeks.

- Establish a written policy for contract and financial management that includes the following:

  + A clear message to all that I am the only one who is authorized to sign contracts and commit the organization to future payments. This needs to not only be communicated to the staff but also to vendors and business partners.

  + All contracts must go through the contract manager. I only sign contracts that are presented to me with a summary sheet by that person. I typically have two meetings per week with this person to review and sign contracts. That's important because you don't want to inject unnecessary delays.

- Conduct a monthly budget review with the CFO (remember the importance of transparency and building trust-based relationships).

Taking full control also gives you the ability to influence where the highest proportions of the budget are flowing. For example, as mentioned earlier, I like to ensure that the training budget gets one of, if not the, highest levels of expenditure because I believe strongly in investing in people.

Service Request Evaluation Process

When someone in your organization has an idea or develops a need for a new IT-related project, it is the easiest thing in the world to instantly agree and add it to the bottom of your ever-growing list of "ongoing" projects. But if you'll recall, one of our goals is to get away from the trap of having 100+ projects in the pipeline because this is inefficient and makes your department appear to be slow and lumbering.

An alternative approach is to set up a system with so many hurdles that most people will give up long before they get to the end of the process. This is effective but is transparently hostile and gives off totally the wrong impression.

The trick is to create criteria that allows requests to be rejected, without making the applicant feel like you were just looking for a reason to say "no." I achieve this by using a Service Request Evaluation Process that assesses and prioritizes requests, while also – and this is the critical component – providing resources that help people make their case.

Below is a flowchart that I use to explain this process to the IT team and to our contacts in the business and clinical departments. This is critical so I would like to help you clearly understand the key steps in the process.

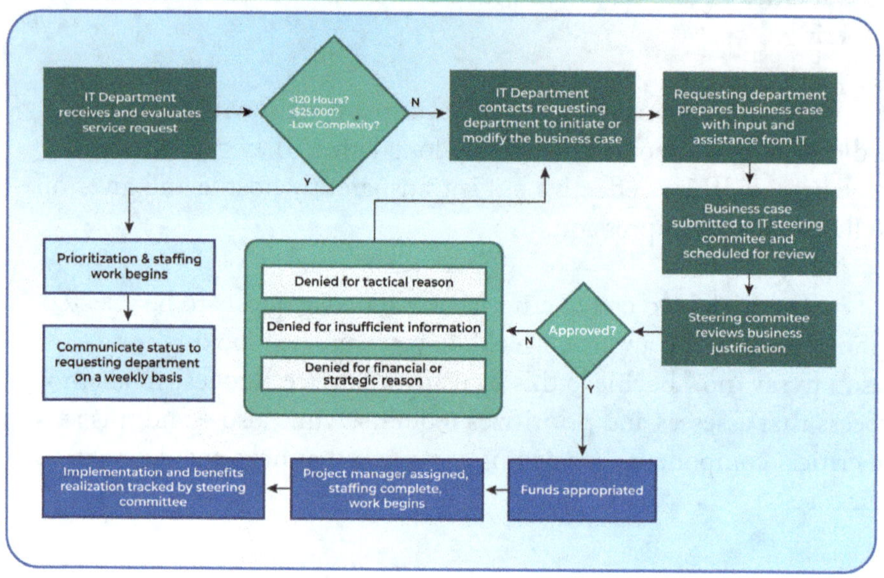

Figure 8.1 Service Request (Work Order)
Submission and Evaluation Process

Step One: Service Request Application

The applicant completes an application form explaining their need, the solution they would like to be created or purchased, and the reason they believe this is the best solution. For example, let's say the cardiology department meets and they establish that their PACS system is coming to the end of its life and needs replacing. If I'm the CIO at this organization I've already given them a head start because one of my IT team members attends their department meetings (you'll discover more on this strategy in the chapter on Governance).

Step Two: IT Department Evaluation

The application is reviewed. If the IT department believes the issue can be solved with a simpler or existing solution, this is communicated to the applicant. However, if the service request has merit, it is assessed against a number of criteria.

Step Three: Criteria Consideration

The designated criteria is designed to allow the IT department to decide if the service request can be implemented quickly and easily, or if it needs further consideration. For example, in the past, I've used a criterion based on time, cost, and complexity. Anything under 120 hours of work AND under $25,000 in cost AND of low complexity, can be accepted, prioritized, and assigned staff.

If, however, the application fails even one of these criteria, it needs to be escalated for a more detailed review.

Step Four: Business Case Creation

If the service request fails one or more of the criteria, the applicant is informed that their application has merit but that it needs further review because of the time, cost, or complexity involved. This requires a detailed business case document to be created and a member of the IT project management team, who has been trained in this process, is assigned to assist them. This pairing up is crucial because it removes any suggestion that unnecessary obstacles are being placed in the way of the applicant just to deter them.

Step Five: Steering Committee Review

Once the business case document has been completed, it is presented to the Business or Clinical steering committee, as appropriate (committee creation and governance will be discussed in more detail in the next chapter).

If the service request is approved by the steering committee, it's then taken forward for funding and project initiation. A project manager is officially assigned, and resources are committed to the project. It is important to note, there are instances when multiple projects are approved. For example, ten clinical projects may be approved after undergoing their respective review process. In this instance, the steering committee will apply an additional layer of prioritization for the projects in order to meet the available resources. In the additional review, the steering committee will analyze all the approved projects in four categories including: "Patient or Regulatory Requirement" (yes/no), "Strategic Alignment to Organization Goals" (yes/no), "Potential Additional Value to Organization" (high/medium/low), and "Resources Needed" (high/medium/low). Utilizing these scales, the Steering Committee can then further help prioritize the execution of all projects in the case of multiple approvals.

If, however, the service request is not approved, the request should not simply be rejected. Rather it should be returned to the original applicant with the specific reasons. You may even, for instance, describe the result as something like, "Not Ready for Approval" rather than simply "Denied" or "Rejected." As depicted in the diagram, the obstacle could be tactical reasons, insufficient information, financial reasons, and so on. The important thing is that the applicant is made aware of the reasons for the outcome and given the opportunity to modify the business case so it can be reviewed again at a later date.

The applicant may decide that there isn't any way to resolve the issue at this time, but it puts the decision back into their hands over whether to keep pushing, look for an alternative idea, or to let the request go for the time being.

Regardless of the approval process, once the budget has been allocated, you're responsible for managing it.

Be Accountable for Your Expenditures

You're going to achieve some amazing wins over the next few years, but some of your initiatives are going to require expenditure. If you want to avoid battles over funding, as well as the headache of going over budget and being asked to axe projects or even staff, you need to take full control of your budget.

This is going to take discipline on your part, but it's also going to take discipline on the part of your team members. They need to understand that every "yes" in one area, likely means a "no" in another area.

Training your team to think through cost-based decisions and understand how to make a business case for every project is a valuable undertaking and will ultimately give you the flexibility to channel funds to where they can provide the most benefit. Not just for you and your colleagues, but ultimately your patients and their families.

This is just a brief discussion of how you and your team are going to establish a financial and contract management discipline and associated processes. Be sure to work with your organization's finance organization to get the appropriate level of support and cooperation for your approach within the IT organization. That is a valuable partnership to foster that will yield great dividends in the future.

To-Do List: Part Seven
(Your 90-Day CIO Strategy Overview)

☐   **Task #1** – Establish a small Finance and Contracts Management team within your department that cares for contracts and financial management, and that allows you to review and give final approval on any future contracts.

☐   **Task #2** - Communicate the new approach to all members of your team, vendors, and partners.

☐   **Task #3** – Schedule a monthly budget review with the CFO.

☐   **Task #4** – Create a Service Request Evaluation Process. This should include criteria against which applications can be reviewed to decide when a more detailed business case is necessary. You will also need to train some of your IT team to be able to assist with the creation of a business case.

BUSINESS CASE SAMPLE: Cardiology PACS Replacement

The following business case sample is based on a real submission that was submitted to the IT department during one of my previous CIO tenures. Some details, including dates, have been fictionalized to maintain anonymity, but the purpose of including this example is to give you an idea of how detailed these submissions should be, and also why it's critical to supply a trained member of your team to assist in the creation of the document. You need this high level of information to make informed decisions, but it's unreasonable to expect every department to have the capabilities of producing a document with this level of detail.

Text in italics are additional comments I've added.

Cardiology PACS Replacement

Business Case

Date Submitted: August 24, 2023

I.   <u>Project Information</u>

Project Name:

Cardiology PACS

Project Description:

Selection and implementation of a new vendor-supplied Cardiology PACS system is considered the primary focus of this presentation. The urgency to address this issue is based on existing software end-of life and support. PACS System replacement is the first of a multi-phase endeavor replacing the disparate Cardiology system assets with a single-vendor set of solutions. By implementing these systems, there will be a marked improvement in the quality of patient care by providing physicians easy access to comprehensive clinical information. Patient safety is enhanced by having one point of entry to patient records that ties together information and imaging from multiple source systems, leading to optimal decision making at the point of care.

(Note that the most important reason why the request is being made – patient care – is stated clearly at the outset.)

PACS System performance and vendor support of the ALPHA system has been inconsistent since BETA was assumed by GAMMA. Dissatisfaction with vendor support has been registered with GAMMA but performance has not lived up to our expectations and thereby the system is viewed as less-than reliable. This places undue concern and constraints on clinical providers using the system at the most inopportune times. The current ALPHA Cardiovascular software is reaching end of life (support) on March 31, 2024.

(Dates and deadlines are critical if the submission is to be treated with due urgency.)

This project is in support of Cardiology's Quality and Financial initiatives. Quality life-saving diagnostic services and reporting must be maintained, and timely financial reimbursement cannot be interrupted.

(And it never hurts to reference the financial imperatives.)

Hardware support provided by GAMMA vendor is also lapsing. DELTA Information Technology Services will support the workstation and server hardware as long as parts supplies are available and/or until a replacement system solution is available.

Project Scope Definition:

At a high level, implementation of a new Cardiology PACS system involves replacing software and hardware, re-establishing connections to acquisition devices used for invasive and non-invasive cardiac procedures, re-affirming or re-designing operational workflows to guarantee operational effectiveness and efficiency, matching up new vendor technologies with existing or enhancing, computing and networking environment, conversion of data and images housed in legacy storage sites, re-establishing connections with external "sending" facilities for image import, and re-establishing communications (interfaces) between our internal sending and receiving systems.

At an elemental level, the technical features of a Cardiology PACS system allow for the most technically advanced measuring cardiac instrumentation and calculations, imagery enhancement and delivery to clinical providers.

The project scope includes submitting a request for information and proposal to Cardiology health solutions software vendors and selecting a vendor for the hospital. The vendor must present their suite of products covering PACS, hemo-dynamics, Interventional Cardiology, Non-Invasive Cardiology (Nuclear Cardiology, Echocardiography) and Electrophysiology. This task began in June of 2023 and is ongoing with expected completion in October 2023 and selection of a new vendor. Contract negotiations are expected to begin shortly afterward, with a thorough contract review with IT, Cardiology, Materials Management and Legal Council.

Implementation tasks may begin as early as fall of 2023.

Further, consideration is being given to cardiology solutions in Cardiology areas for possible enterprise-level expansion with a single vendor solution.

(This is a good summary and allows for a more accurate assessment of the funds and staffing that will be required.)

——

Desired Start Date: July 1, 2023
Expected End Date: December 31, 2023

Name of Project Sponsor: Jane Doe, VP Cardiology

Business Unit: Hospital
Department: Cardiology

Project's Support for Business Strategy:

Cardiology PACs and its clinical applications will support the integration of services and expertise across the continuum of care and allow the hospital to leverage the best practices available in the Division of Cardiology. Having a common system will not only protect the organizations from regulatory threats but support our balance scorecard initiatives.

Project's Support for Mission and Vision:

In support of the hospital's mission and vision, an integrated Cardiology PACs system supports the core strategies of a unified operating environment, care coordination, and clinical integration.

A core focus of this implementation is to standardize best practices throughout Cardiology while providing a single clinical experience regardless of location. This will not only support future and current collaborations for safe, effective patient care, but will afford the flexibility to staff and patients in accessing their health information wherever they are being treated in the continuum of care.

The system selection focuses heavily on clinical staff utilization of the system and their input is driving the selection process. Our focus is to be as inclusive as possible, understanding we are choosing what will become the only portal users will have to access Cardiology PACs information.

(A useful requirement for these business cases is for the author to explain how this project will help further the organization's mission statement or other critical initiatives.)

II. Benefits

The proposed clinical integration amongst the entities of Cardiology will support the initiatives of a unified operating environment and a coordinated care model. By drawing on the expertise across our diverse system in both clinical practice and compliance in Cardiology interventional and diagnostic care, Cardiology will position itself to mitigate risk and take advantage of best practice.

(The "Benefits" section will often be the longest and most detailed part of the business case. The author needs to make a strong and exhaustive case, not just for why it is valuable, but why it is potentially more critical than other projects that may be vying for attention.)

- **Financial Benefits: Increased Revenue or Decreased Costs**

This project is in support of the Division of Cardiology Service Excellence, Quality, and Financial scorecard pillars. Service Excellence: improvement in the coordination of care beginning with the referring physician community; Quality: life-saving diagnostic services and reporting must be maintained; Financial: timely financial reimbursement cannot be interrupted.

Selection and implementation of a new vendor-supplied Cardiology PACS system is considered the primary focus due to upcoming software end-of life. It is the first of a multi-phase endeavor replacing cardiology system assets with a single-vendor set of solutions. Cardiology expects to replace the hemo-dynamic system in rapid fashion soon after PACS implementation.

There is an expected decrease of administrative costs including eliminating transcription and the expense associated with sending copies of reports to EPSILON for processing. There will also be a decrease in the turnaround time of report generation which will result in timely billing and reimbursement of procedures.

- **CMS Reporting Requirements**

Automation of required reporting to national databases that interface with CMS for reporting Core Measures, which will potentially impact reimbursement in 2025.

- **Improved Patient Quality**

The proposed system will allow information to be entered once and used throughout the system and, by leveraging best practices, create a flow that makes sense to providers. More importantly, the ability to gather and refer to real-time clinical data either past or present will affect patient outcomes and satisfaction.

- **Improved Employee Productivity**

The primary goal of our electronic system is to provide our employees with the information they need, in the format they need it, and at the time they need it. This is true of both clinical and business departments. Further, guided work lists, reminders, and clinical alerts will support employee job functions and reduce lost work and rework. See below for improved productivity in a downtime situation.

- **Improved Asset Management**

The automated report generation system will allow for a decrease in clerical work that may result in decrease of administrative costs associated with report generation.

The ability to move Cardiology to a virtualized server environment will be a savings to IT in both asset and time management, by reducing hard assets, required space, and technician time. Additionally, in the virtualized server environment, documented annual downtime has been dramatically reduced, in some cases from 2-3 days to 8-12 hours. Back-up server sites are not needed in the virtual environment, therefore eliminating redundancy cost. Efficiencies are gained since test environments and application refreshments can occur without downtime.

- **Financial Benefits Projection**

	FY2023	FY2024	FY2025	FY2026	FY2027	FY2028	FY2029
Initial Cost		$850,000	$650,000				
Annual depreciation		$214,086	$214,086	$214,086	$214,086	$214,086	$214,086

Intangible Benefits:

(A business outline can be provided with pre-populated headings to nudge the author into digging deeper. For example, the author may not think about how the project might improve employee morale until they're specifically prompted.)

- ## Image of the Organization

The new PACS and report generation system will improve the overall image of the hospital and Cardiology by providing reliable and timely results and access to patient information that will support the continuum of care and provide an improved patient experience. As we further integrate cardiac clinical practices, access to patient data will be critical to the success of this collaborative effort.

- ## Service to the (Patient) Communities

These new technologies will position our organization to provide providers with better access to health information and support continuity of care activities between providers. Improved coordination of care with referring medical providers will also benefit patients and clients of our system.

- ## Employees Morale

Employees will appreciate the ability to access the medical record throughout our system, VPN, and various portal applications. This will reduce the time searching for 'charts', diagnostic data found in other systems within Cardiology, or other related information and create an on-demand health information service. We expect marked improvement in compliance, productivity, and a reduction in redundancy.

- ## Patient Satisfaction

Patient satisfaction will be enhanced by improved responsiveness, reduced redundancy, and improved clinical decision making. Clinical documentation is available and legible at the point of care further enhancing client trust and satisfaction.

- **Meet Regulatory Compliance**

The current systems in place within Cardiology rely on staff memory, manual audit, or retroactive reporting to ensure compliance. The proposed system, through its integrated reminder and alerting systems, will present the user with a work list required to maintain regulatory compliance. If these lists and reminders are ignored, they are automatically escalated through a pre-approved hierarchy to clinical and fiscal leadership.

- **Improve Decisions (Clinical and/or administrative)**

The new system report generation software will allow for timely communication of results to referring physicians that will allow for a more timely decision making of care and treatment.

III. <u>Project Costs</u>

(Summary provided below. Typically, a financials spreadsheet with all the associated costs accompanies the business case. The finance team along with the vendor are usually a good source for this information.)

	FY23	FY24	FY25	FY26	FY27	FY28	Total
Licenses							
Implementation							
Hardware							
Subtotal							
Staffing							
Capital		$850,000	$650,000				
Capital Staffing							
Operating Staffing							
Maintenance			$160,796	$270,000	$270,000	$270,000	
Total Project		$850,000	$810,796	$270,000	$270,000	$270,000	$2,470,796

IV.   <u>Project Risk</u>

(This section considers both sides of the risk; risks as a consequence of carrying out the project, and risks of NOT carrying out the project.)

System performance and vendor support of the ALPHA system has been inconsistent. Dissatisfaction with vendor support has been registered. Current ALPHA Cardiovascular software is reaching end of life (support) on March 31, 2024.

Hardware support is also lapsing on vendor supplied workstations. Information Technology Services will continue support of hardware (workstations and servers) as permitted through available part supplies until a replacement solution is available.

Current GAMMA imaging servers are exhibiting multiple component failures; vendor not providing hardware support services.

V.   <u>Preliminary Project Organization</u>

The project will be led by N. Monk. The project team will consist of a project manager, lead clinical application specialist, vendor project leader, and vendor implementation lead. This core team will report to the Steering Committee which is comprised of the core executives in the hospital.

VI.   <u>Additional Information</u>

This solution is scalable as other imaging entities are added to SHC.

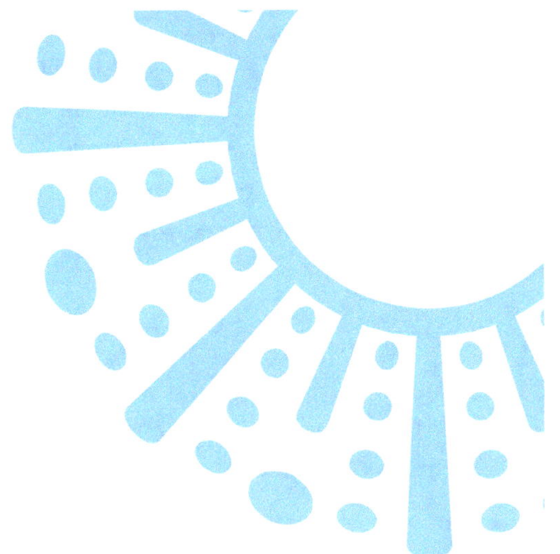

CHAPTER NINE:

Governance – Continuing the Drive towards High Performance

I once arrived at a new organization and the leadership team, with the best of intentions, decided to help me out in advance by disbanding the Project Management Office (PMO). There had been some issues with my predecessor, and they had let him go along with the head of the PMO. And as part of that liability, the PMO was completely removed. The perceived wisdom was that this particular team was ineffective and that removing this resource would help streamline things for me when I arrived.

Without being critical or judgmental, I quickly let them know that I absolutely needed a project management team and that we should put a new department in place as soon as possible. The simple fact is that good governance is impossible without a PMO because you need that team of people who can oversee projects, track their development, and make sure they're proceeding correctly and efficiently.

I took a former CIO from one of the organization's divisions and named him the head of the new PMO. He was perfect for this role because he was well respected and had that kind of brain and personality that really thrived on keeping things organized. He took the new appointment really seriously and between us we added more people to his team until we had a solid department.

With the PMO team intact again, we arranged for them to receive proper training and certification in project management. We made a deal with a local university and arranged for the entire team to receive a project management curriculum and proper qualifications at the end of it.

In just a short time the department flourished, and projects began being delivered on time, while also adding real value to the organization. I'm still in touch with some of the people there and even to this day, their PMO is one of the strongest teams at that organization. They've successfully led some massive projects from start to finish, and they should be immensely proud of what they've achieved.

What this illustrates is that when governance fails it has little to do with the people, or the concept of governance, and everything to do with proper training and organization. A high-performing healthcare organization uses a governance model at all levels, and it's structured in a way that ensures each stage of development is properly managed, that the work being completed is properly tracked and measured, and that everyone knows exactly who is responsible for every piece of the puzzle.

Governance is The Glue

The above illustration is also an example of how common it is for a CIO to fail to put together a proper governance model. The sad truth is that too many organizations, even under the watch of an experienced CIO, are mainly relying on an ad hoc structure where too many projects are taken on at once, and priority is based on whatever individuals in different positions feel on a given day.

It's even possible to have dozens of departments and committees but still be essentially operating in a haphazard fashion if the departments don't connect properly and if there isn't a clear structure for making consistent decisions.

Tell me if this sounds familiar…

If a senior person in your organization, with a forceful personality, decides one day that, in their opinion, a particular project should be the number one priority, could they just make it happen? Could they go to key people in various departments, pull rank, and yank them off their existing projects to focus on this new idea? All without any committee discussion, without any business case preparation or proper costing?

Be honest with yourself. Even if that exact scenario hasn't played itself out, have you witnessed something similar? Or are you aware that, at the very least, it COULD happen?

If so, don't worry, you're in good company. But you need to put a structure in place that makes it virtually impossible for this to happen.

This near certainty comes from the fact that we've established a strong foundation that will allow us to build towards a high-performance organization, the final stage is governance. Get this right, and everything you've created – the culture, the systems, the guiding principles – will run like clockwork with virtually no slippages or blockages. Get this wrong and you'll experience symptoms such as:

+ Slow decision-making

+ Senior management being unclear on who is in charge of specific areas.

+ Projects behind schedule and over budget.

+ A tendency to bring in expensive consultants or even outsource as a desperate measure to get things back on track.

+ Constant shuffling of governance practices and leadership.

The moment you start to see evidence of any of these problems – and you might recognize some already – the problem is usually related to a lack of well-organized governance.

Simply put, governance is the glue that holds everything together and ensures everyone keeps moving in the same direction. If you want a more specific description, my preferred definition is…

Governance: Identifies the interactions among the levels of authority, the decision-making process by these authorities, and who will be accountable for the performance and achievements of the expected results.

There are many other definitions of governance out there, but they mostly point to the same key factor – accountability. Without a clear understanding of who is responsible for each element of any process, you're likely to see projects stall, disappear down dead ends, or get locked into cycles of endless bureaucracy where no one wants to or is able to make a decision.

When this happens, what eventually results, is that the accountability lands on your doorstep. Quite right too, but we're not going to resolve these issues by trying to be the casting vote on every project decision.

Your final step in your 90-day journey is to define your governance model and, as always, to get buy-in from everybody involved.

This is What Success Looks Like

Begin by creating your own definition of governance. Feel free to steal the one above or create something similar that better fits your specific organization. Next, create a series of success factors against which your governance model can be measured. In other words, performance metrics and qualities that your governance teams should be reaching. They may look something like this:

- ✦ Management involved at all levels across the entire organization.

- ✦ Clearly defined decision-making process.

- ✦ Decisions being made with the entire organization in mind… not just a specific person or department.

- ✦ Provision for exception handling when necessary.

- ✦ Appropriate representation of all parts of the organization.

- ✦ Ownership and accountability clearly assigned.

- ✦ Transparency at all levels.

- ✦ Governance teams given freedom to evolve along with your organization's maturity.

Whatever the precise model you create, aim to establish something that gives you the organizational structure you are aiming for, that drives the proper implementation of new technologies, allows you the flexibility to support a changing and evolving environment, and supports the learning and development of your staff.

For added clarity, create a visual representation of the overall model that will help you educate your teams on how things are going to work from this point forward. Below is the overall governance model that I use as a template when I arrive at a new organization.

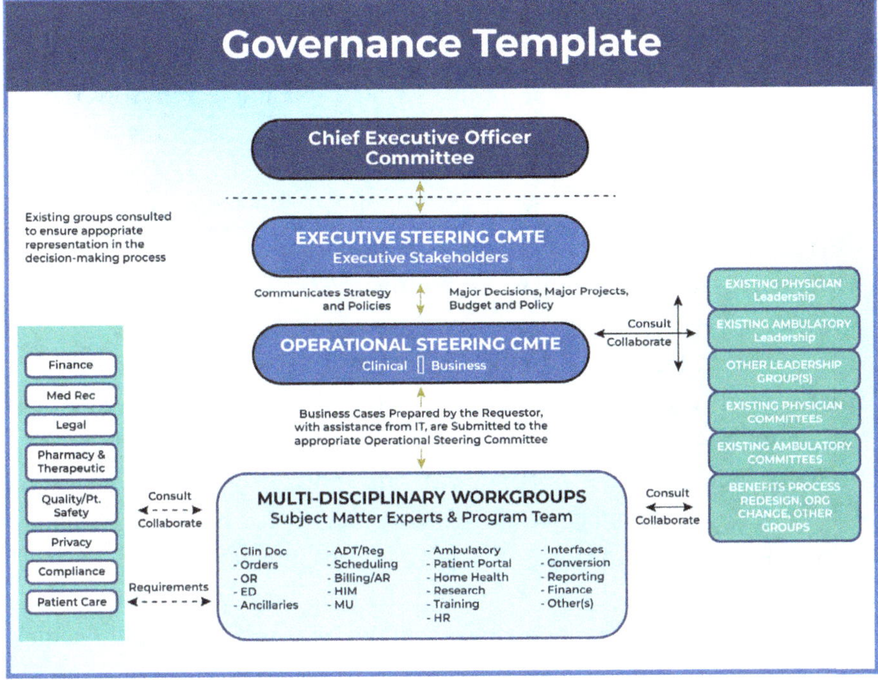

Figure 9.1. Sample Governance Model

The columns on the far left and far right are all the existing committees, groups and departments that likely already exist within your healthcare organization. If one of these groups has an IT need, this is communicated to one or more of the multi-disciplinary workgroups (illustrated in the bottom middle of the diagram) and dialogue is carried out to establish the feasibility and necessity of the recommendation.

If it's decided that there is a strong business case, the project starts to move up the chain. First to the Operational Steering Committee who will consider the clinical and financial implications of the project. Then if it's approved but is an expensive or time-consuming endeavor, it moves up to the Executive Steering Committee. Finally, if the project still has the green light but is a major, major expense, it moves up to the top of the organization, the CEO Committee (or, as I prefer to call it, the CEO Council).

But here's the real secret to making this work…

You're going to assign one of your IT team as a liaison or primary point of contact to every existing committee and workgroup. Essentially, in the same way that we took advantage of existing training programs and regular meetings to slide in some cybersecurity training, you're going to piggyback onto all the existing committees so that, when there's an IT need, you have someone in place to assist.

If this sounds a little bit like you're creating a network of spies… well… maybe there is a little bit of that – part of the role of the IT members you place in each of the committees or workgroups is there to make sure that people don't sidestep your governance system – but the key difference is that this isn't an adversarial strategy. The person assigned to, for example, the Patient Care committee is going to attend their meetings and be kept in the loop with what's happening in that area of the organization so that, when an IT need is identified, your IT person can assist them with performing the research, consulting with the appropriate workgroups, and creating the business proposal that is sent up to the Operational Steering Committee.

In fact, when you're operating at a high-performance level, your IT placements can and should be proactive in identifying the committees' needs and making recommendations as to how they can be addressed. Instead of waiting for people to come to you, you're going to go to them. I cannot overstate what a difference this makes in the long run, not just in ensuring that the governance structure is followed, but in ensuring the right projects are presented in the right way, so that what your organization needs most to improve the quality of your staff's work and the end result for patients are what's delivered. We must get away from this idea that IT is a department of order-takers;

that we just sit around waiting for people to come to us with a need or
a problem.

Everyone has their own learning style. But a visual model of
how projects are going to be governed seems to be perfect for quickly
helping everyone see that things are going to be different from how
they used to be. Everything is going to be managed and delivered in
an engaging and disciplined way, and there's no way for anyone to hide
from the outcomes of their work.

It won't surprise you to learn that not everyone responds
positively to this significant level of change. You may hear some
grumbling about things becoming too bureaucratic, or that this new
method will slow things down. What they usually mean is that the
quick and shoddy method they've been coasting along with is in
danger of being dissolved, and this isn't going to sit well with some
people.

Either that or they may have worked hard to create special
relationships with certain managers or departments that previously
allowed them to get their requests prioritized. This new model is
going to level the playing field and remove any meritocracies that have
developed.

It's important that you handle negative reactions swiftly so
they don't spread, but also trust that most people will recognize why
sometimes going a little slower in some places allows everyone to
actually move faster. Make it clear that this model is designed to drive
productivity increases and ensure that everyone can stay focused on the
right things at the right time.

The Goals are The Same

There can be many types, levels, and linkages of governance within an organization. You may need, or already have, teams that govern some of the following areas:

+ Finance

+ Medical Records

+ Legal

+ Pharmacy and Therapeutics

+ Quality and Patient Safety

+ Privacy

+ Compliance

+ Patient Care

+ Physicians

+ Ambulatory

+ IT department

+ Project management

+ Portfolio/Program

+ Data

In all cases, governance is not strictly a control mechanism, but it is a way to manage, guide, track progress, facilitate progress, and achieve the expected results. For example, let's look at components of IT department governance – specifically the Service Request Evaluation Process described in the previous chapter (Figure 8.1).

Remember that in this process, simple requests of less than 120 hours and less than $25,000 in cost and low level of complexity are responded to quickly. I usually set up a pool of staff members who are dedicated to work on these quick-order items. The more complex requests need to go through a business case process that is guided by the project managers on the team. This is why it's so critical to have a fully staffed and strong project management office.

What makes this process so outstanding is that every loop is inherently closed. Projects can't disappear down cul-de-sacs or wind up floating around endlessly without any decisions being made. The closest a service request could get to this latter scenario is if a business case is rejected and then resubmitted. But even then, a resubmission would require substantial changes and would only repeat the loop if the interested party is willing to put the time in to make the business case more viable; essentially, this makes the loop self-limiting.

Your goal should be to create flow charts such as this one for every governance department you create. For example, here's a committee I create for the Security Oversight Group (SOG) at all of my organizations.

Responsibilities	Participants
• Responsible for consistency of decisions across all business areas related to information security and privacy. • Review security and privacy incidents for regulatory and information risk management. • Review and discuss cybersecurity challanges and risk to the health system. • Responsible for authorizing the development and implementation of information Security polices, standards, procedures and guidelines. • Review and approve proposed strategic initiatives to ensure they align with system enterprise strategies and methodologies.	- Chief Information Officer - Chief Legal Officer & Privacy Officer - Chief Human Resources Officer - VP Internal Audit - VP Applications - Chief Information Security Officer - Manager Internal Audit - Deputy Counsel Legal Officers - Others (Ad-Hoc as Needed)

Figure 9.2. Security Oversight Group
Responsibilities and Participants

A flow chart for this committee may be similar, although somewhat simpler, than the Service Request process, in that it creates a process for departments to report security incidents or concerns, to consult with the workgroups as required, and then to present recommended actions for the above committee to review.

It will take time to create any missing committees, to assign an IT team member to each committee and department, and to help everyone involved understand the importance of carrying out the work in this fashion. So, your main objective during your first 90 days is to identify the groups that need to be set up, select the participants, itemize their responsibilities and, if possible, create a flow chart that determines how information is gathered and communicated to them by the rest of the organization.

The Final Piece of The Puzzle

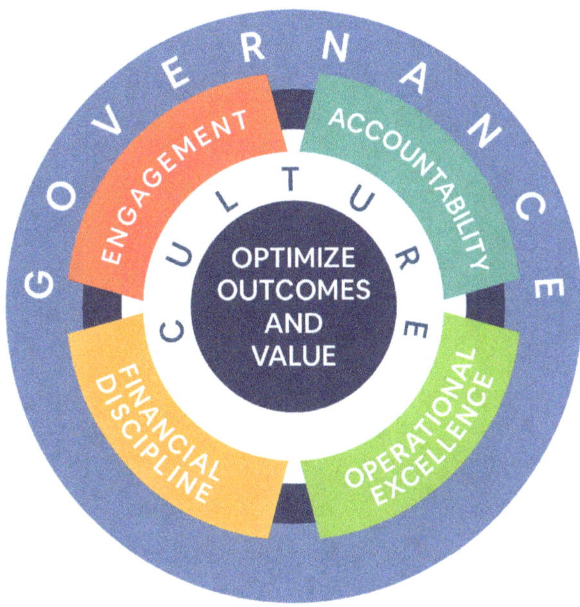

Figure 10.1. The 90 Day CIO Model ©

It has been some time, maybe 90 days, since we first considered the 90-Day CIO Model Framework, but hopefully by this point you can see why Governance is the discipline that wraps around everything else. Individually, each element is powerfully transformative, but organizations of all sizes – especially those of the size typical to healthcare businesses – have a tendency to trend back into old habits if you don't find a way to lock new processes in place. Good governance models are what will allow you to glue all your hard work together and keep everybody on track with their new processes, methodologies and systems.

Without a strong governance system in place, every time something out of the ordinary occurs, or every time some new IT system is considered, everyone just scrambles and does the best they can to react quickly and accurately. But inevitably this slows down the process, people retreat into their cliques, and different priorities butt heads leaving progress in limbo.

In contrast, good governance means that almost no decision-making is required when a new scenario presents itself – at least through the early stages of the process. Your flow charts and processes will ensure everyone knows who is required to do what, who is managing the outcome, and how the resolution is measured for efficacy.

At one of the organizations I worked for, when I first arrived, there was little to no proper governance in place. And it was hard to change that mindset because there were unions who held a lot of the power over what could and couldn't be changed. It was like working with one hand tied behind my back.

I started out by scheduling monthly meetings, which traditionally never happened. I used those meetings to share my strategic plans with everyone and helped them to see the benefits they could enjoy if we all pulled in the same direction. It was hard to get people engaged in what we were doing so, it was a small token, but I started buying a $25 gift card out of my own money and gifting it to an "employee of the month" (make sure you speak to your HR department before trying anything like this) at each meeting. It was a small gesture, but it helped people to look forward to and be interested in coming together as a team.

As I mentioned earlier, in this organization, I had no budget to build a cybersecurity team, so I needed people to volunteer to participate on top of their regular duties. It would have been impossible to get enough people on board without getting people to embrace the ideals of accountability and team spirit.

Depending on the type of healthcare (and non-healthcare) organization you're at, and the historic challenges you may be facing, some elements of your journey are going to be easier than others. But it is always possible. It might just require some patience and some creative initiatives for getting people to actively participate.

A Principled Organization

It's been said that principles are superior to laws because it takes only a handful of principles, properly upheld, to achieve the same end as any number of laws. Not to get religious on you, but the classic example is Jesus Christ reducing the hundreds of edicts found in Israelite law and the Ten Commandments to simply love God and love your neighbor. In the same way, when the principles you put in place at your healthcare organization are embraced and followed by your colleagues, decisions can be made faster and with greater accuracy and consistency than attempting to account for every possible scenario.

The guiding principles that we establish through the improvements to the culture, the transparent communication policies, and the well-structured governance committees, should resonate throughout all of your departments and be felt by the physicians, the administrators, and the patients and their families.

The vision is to develop a committed high-performance organization, with engaged team members who are constantly learning and leading, to advance the strategy of your healthcare organization and the communities we serve.

You can't achieve all of this in 90 days, and I don't suggest you try. But what you accomplish in this timeframe, if carried out in a committed, confident, determined manner, can set the stage for several years of improvements in all areas of your organization.

Remember to have faith in yourself and those around you, have patience in abundance and volunteer discretionary effort at all times. This is the winning combination. I wish you every success!

To-Do List: Part Eight
(Your 90-Day CIO Strategy Overview)

☐   **Task #1** – Create your own definition of governance that will serve as your "North Star."

☐   **Task #2** – Create a list of success factors that can be used to measure performance of the committees you form.

☐   **Task #3** – Design a visual representation of your overall governance model to help communicate your vision.

☐   **Task #4** – Create any missing committees, select the participants, and itemize their responsibilities.

☐   **Task #5** – Create a flow-chart for each governance committee so you can be certain there are no dead-ends or time-wasting loops.

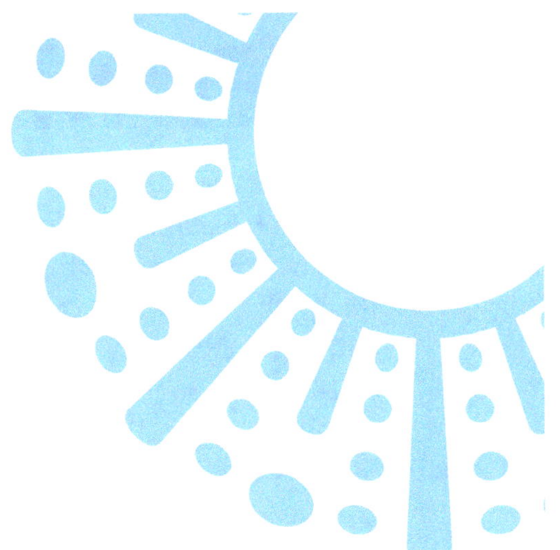

CHAPTER TEN:

The 90-Day Plan and Final Words from a Fellow CIO

We have ended each of the chapters with a task list that will assist you in creating your 90-day plan. Here is a consolidated plan broken down into 30-days segments. Ideally, you will use eighty percent of this plan as suggested but each one of your organizations is different and you are all at different stages of maturity. Therefore, use this as a guide to tailor the plan that best fits you and your organization.

+ Place the 90-Day CIO Strategy and the IT Triple Aim somewhere where you'll see it multiple times a day. Regularly review it so that your primary targets become burned into your brain. Look for opportunities and share these with your colleagues.

+ Set your five (or ten) year targets based on what you need to achieve and then use these to brainstorm a list of tangible milestones. With the engagement and assistance of others, arrange these targets and milestones in order of priority.

+ Put together a rough schedule for the next 90 days that allows room for reviewing, planning, and then executing your plans.

+ Write out a list of the skills and qualities that will be essential to creating your desired culture, and rate yourself on each. Ask other trusted colleagues to rate you and look for gaps in your abilities and attitudes that need improvement.

+ Arrange, within the next 90 days, to have a one-on-one meeting with every executive at your organization to share with them your plans. Start with senior management and work your way down.

+ Establish a Daily Service Review call/meeting with your
leadership team to be completed no later than 8am each
morning. During the role-call, require all participants to
answer the following, or similar, questions.

  - What have you accomplished (since yesterday's call)?
  - What do you intend to accomplish today?
  - What obstacles are you facing and what do you need
    to overcome them?

+ Acquire a list of vendors, ordered from high to low in
terms of annual spend. Proactively look for opportunities to
streamline, remove or bring the service inhouse.

+ Check what your cyber insurance policy covers and consider
whether it is adequate for your needs.

+ Audit your hardware and software cyber security defenses
and identify areas of weakness or that haven't been upgraded
for some time.

+ Review your service management suite of tools and make
sure they support the plan. If not, include procurement and
implementation of new tools into your plan.

+ Create an IT finance and contracting team that cares for
contracts and financial management, and that allows you to
review and give final approval on any future contracts.

+ Create your own set of IT Guiding Principles.

+ Share your IT Guiding Principles with your leadership team first and then with the other executives in the organization. Invite them to comment, tweak or add to your framework and content.

+ Write out a list of the social determinants that you believe to be most relevant to the community you care for.

+ Arrange to speak to other department heads within your organization who may be able to provide additional insights in the area of population health management (PHM).

+ If you have a PHM program in your organization or area, contact those responsible and inquire as to how you can support them more fully and even expand their reach. If you don't have a PHM program in your area, speak to people within your organization to make your own list of potential initiatives you could create on your own or assist in creating.

+ Expand the leadership skills assessment exercise across the rest of your leadership team so you can identify training needs. Meet with each person individually to review their results and establish an improvement plan.

+ Review the outside assets, such as consultants, that you're using and consider whether any of it can be scaled back, either now or in the future.

+ Look through your calendar and make a list of how many times you have had meetings with people other than at board level.

+ Create a charter of leadership principles that you want your managers to follow and, if necessary, build some training around them.

+ Identify any disruptive individuals among the leadership team and either coach them or let them go.

+ Create a pact with your leadership team to follow an agreed list of rules of engagement.

+ Identify the individuals most resistant to engaging with these new initiatives. Seek to train and/or encourage them to participate, and if they are unable or unwilling, move them on swiftly, but humanely.

+ Review (or create) your security plan. Share it and obtain feedback from your department heads and make sure it covers the resources and policies you have in place, as well as the projects in development. Share the results with the CEO and the members of the cabinet and make sure that they support all of your ongoing and planned initiatives.

+ Establish your Security Oversight Group and begin the monthly meetings.

+ Create plans that outline how you will respond to any future security breaches.

+ Assess your current processes and map them to ITIL.

+ Develop an ITIL primer for the education and awareness of the entire IT staff.

+ Create a list of success factors that can be used to measure performance of the committees you form.

+ Widen the scope and reach out to organizations and community leaders who may also be able to provide useful insights and recommendations.

+ Once you have a good overall view of the social determinants for your region, consider the data that will help you gain a deeper understanding, the organizations that can help you obtain this data, and the person or persons inside or outside of your organization who can help you and the rest of the leadership team interpret this data and turn it into valuable information for all.

+ Set up a monthly lunch for around a dozen people in your team and invite a different group each month.

+ Schedule a quarterly team-wide call to update everyone on their progress and to commend their efforts.

+ Plan an annual event, involving every employee, which includes presentations from the leadership team, and some fun, team-building activities.

+ Invite your top vendors and service providers to a meeting where you will share your strategic plan with them and seek their assistance in meeting your long-term goals.

+ Plan and schedule regular cyber awareness training. Make sure every member of the organization, regardless of seniority, attends.

+ Carry out regular penetration testing and conduct quarterly phishing exercises. Report the results of these exercises and ensure that the sanctions plan agreed upon is adhered to by all departments, including the termination of those who fail for a third time.

+ Communicate your strategic plan to the leadership team of the organization.

+ Schedule a monthly budget review with the CFO.

+ Create a Service Request Evaluation Process. This should include criteria against which applications can be reviewed to decide when a more detailed business case is necessary. You will also need to train some of your IT team to be able to assist with the creation of a business case document.

+ Design a visual representation of your entire organization to help communicate your vision.

+ Create a flow-chart for each governance committee so you can be certain there are no dead-ends or time-wasting loops.

+ Establish any missing committees, select the participants, and itemize their responsibilities.

Are your 90 days up? If so, I want you to take a moment to reflect on how much you have accomplished in the last three months. I'm a realist so I don't expect you to have ticked off every assignment in every chapter just yet (that doesn't mean you can skip any steps, but you might need a couple of extra weeks to mop up the last few items), but if you've tackled this 90-day strategy with heart and intensity you should be somewhere close. In the appendices you'll find a complete list of every task, so after you've finished reading this chapter, take a moment to review it and identify any steps that remain.

You've done some incredible work that has laid the foundation for moving you from being a reactive CIO, to well on your way to finding operational excellence, with a future goal of eventually reaching the level of high performance. But don't lose sight of the fact that it is just a foundation. The foundation is an essential part of any building, but it's pointless if you don't then build something significant on top of it. Don't rest on your laurels and think that the hard work is done. What happens next may be less complicated because you've already established the strategies that will revolutionize your success as a CIO, but you need to keep zealously pushing to ensure that everyone keeps moving in the right direction and that old, lumbering, and even toxic, practices don't reemerge. For all the hard work you've put into the last 90 days, most of it was essentially planning – now it's time to put everything into practice.

Which is why the final task is to write out your long-term plans. Where do you want to be in 12 months? Where do you want to be in three years? Where do you want to be in five years? And so on. Your plan doesn't have to be set in stone (rigidity is not a helpful quality in the CIO of a healthcare organization), and you will likely have to make adjustments to reflect changes in the business, changes in regulations, changes in society, etc., but you should make a plan anyway and review it at regular intervals to ensure you're staying the course.

But if you need something else to work on in the short-term, focus on your leadership skills. Just because you're confident in your ability to complete the planning stage and drive things forward, this in itself doesn't make you a good leader. You must continue to build a trust-based relationship with the people you work with day in and day out. And you must take the initiative to assess your progress in this regard. Ask a trusted colleague to give you feedback or invite your team to rate your abilities (anonymously, of course) so you can identify areas in which you can improve.

At some point, however, things are going to slot into place, and you will find you have a new challenge. It'll likely happen somewhere in between the operational excellence and the high-performance stage. Your IT team will be firing on all cylinders, and you'll be delivering well above expectations. You'll have developed a great culture where everyone holds themselves accountable, and you'll have executed your strategy exactly as you planned it. You'll have become a highly respected and visible leader in the organization.

And this is when you need to take care not to become a victim of your own success.

Don't ever think that you're perfect because there is no such thing as perfection. Maintain your focus and don't allow yourself or others to fall off the bandwagon just because things are going well. You must strive to become the Chief Humble Officer who keeps their team from becoming overconfident and losing their focus.

The disciplined approach that got you to this point needs to be continued. When you have normal turnover and add new members to your team, quickly mold them into your approach. But do not fall into the trap of intransigence. Remember, you're the change agent and must continue to be so. Show flexibility and agility but don't let it affect the stability of what you've built. Our environment is forever changing, you and your team will need to continue to learn from each other and from everything that you do. That's the essence of the learning organization that you've masterminded.

Perhaps most importantly of all, you need to acknowledge everybody's efforts and celebrate their success at all levels of the organization.

You have done it! Continue to enjoy the ride and to reach the bar regardless of how high it gets.

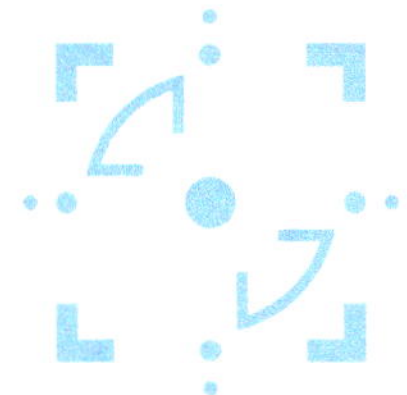

Appendix A:

All Tables and Figures

Figure 1.1 A comparison of outcomes with and without the 90 Day CIO Strategy.

Figure 2.1. The 90 Day CIO Model ©

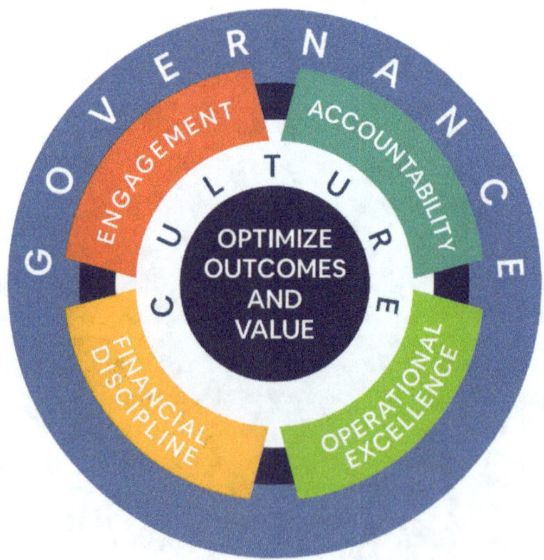

	Personal Assessment	Team Assessment
BASIC SKILLS		
Listening	3	3.2
Communication (via email)	2	2.9
Communication (with peers)	2	2.8
Communication (with reports)	3	3.1
Communication (in small groups)	3	2.9
Communication (in large groups)	3	3.5
Facilitates effective meetings	4	3.1
Effective team leader	3	3.2
Manages work/life balance	4	2.5
Financial management	4	2.5
Strategic thinker	4	3.7
MANAGEMENT SKILLS		
Ability to manage employees	3	2.6
Courageous conversations	3	3.2
Manages difficult issues	3	2.9
Open, honest communication	3	3.3
Holds team accountable	2	3.2
Expectations management	2	2.7
Trusted by employees	3	2.6
Ability to accept and manage change	2	3.1
LEADERSHIP SKILLS		
Perceived as a leader	3	3.4
Discretionary effort	3	2.8
Models high performance	2	3.4
Respects / Leverage separate realities	2	2.7
Curious (but not judgmental)	3	3.1
Holds self-accountable	4	2.1
Acts as a change agent	2	3.6
Supportive of others' efforts	3	3.2

Figure 4.2 Vendor Relationship Matrix.

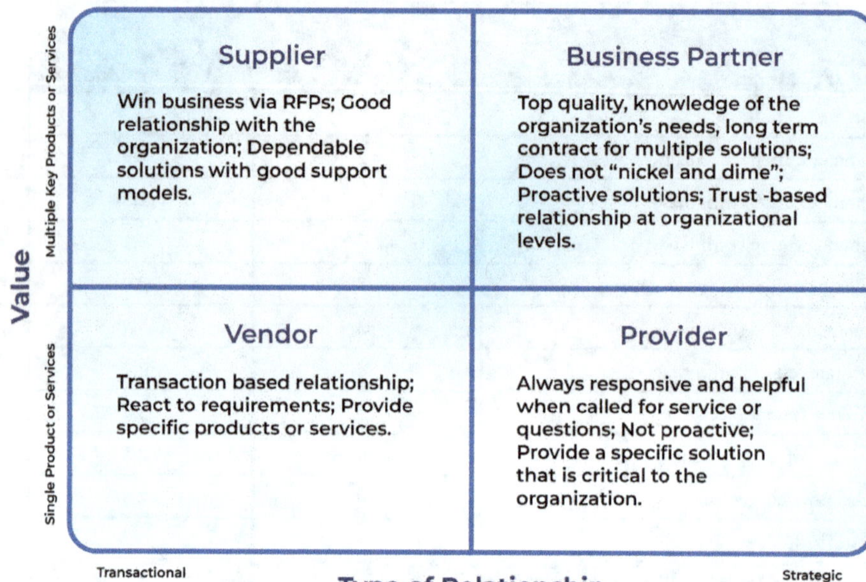

Figure 6.1. 20/20 Security Framework

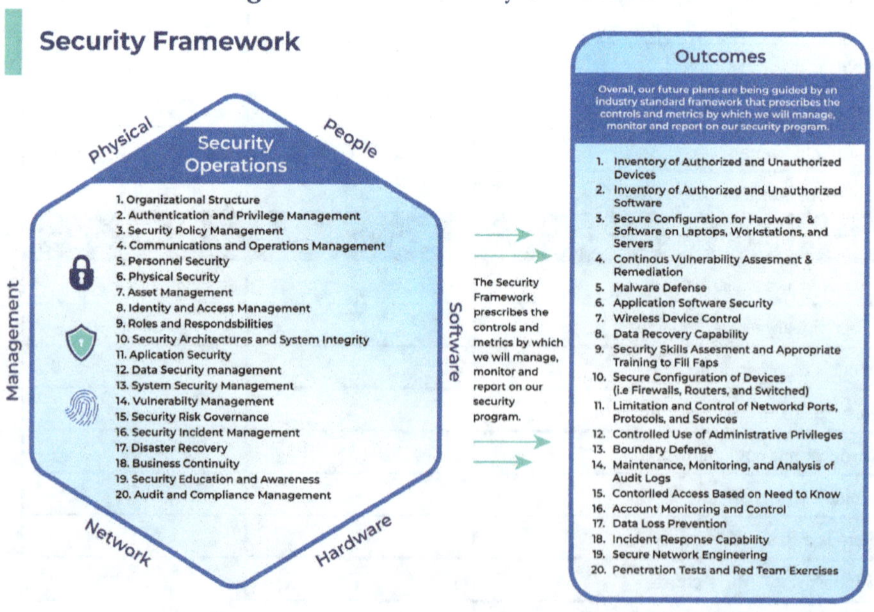

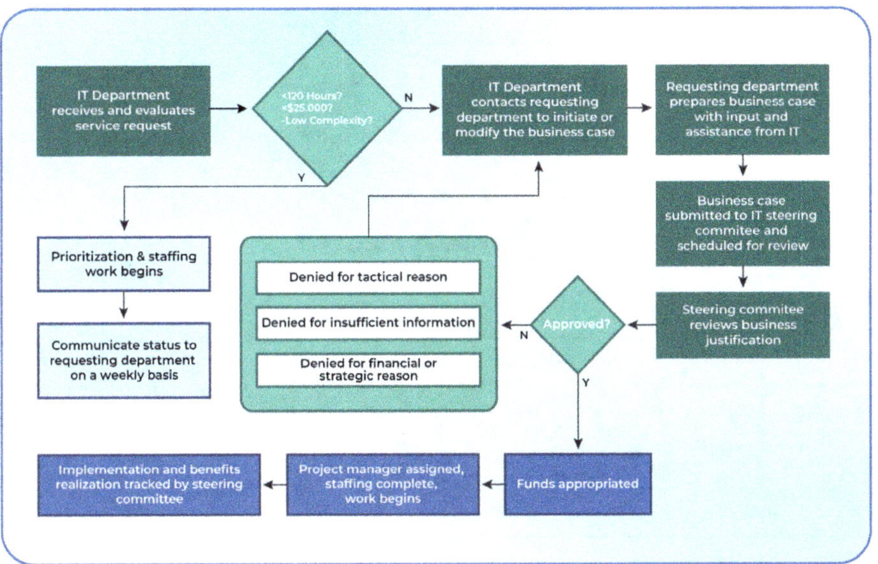

Service Request (Work Order)
Submission and Evaluation Process
IT Department receives and evaluates service request
<120 Hours? <$25.000? -Low Complexity?
N
Y
IT Department contacts requesting department to initiate or modify the business case
Requesting department prepares business case with input and assistance from IT
Business case submitted to IT steering commitee and scheduled for review
Prioritization & staffing work begins
Communicate status to requesting department on a weekly basis
Denied for tactical reason
Denied for insufficient information
Denied for financial or strategic reason
Approved?
N
Y
Steering commitee reviews business justification
Implementation and benefits realization tracked by steering committee
Project manager assigned, staffing complete, work begins
Funds appropriated

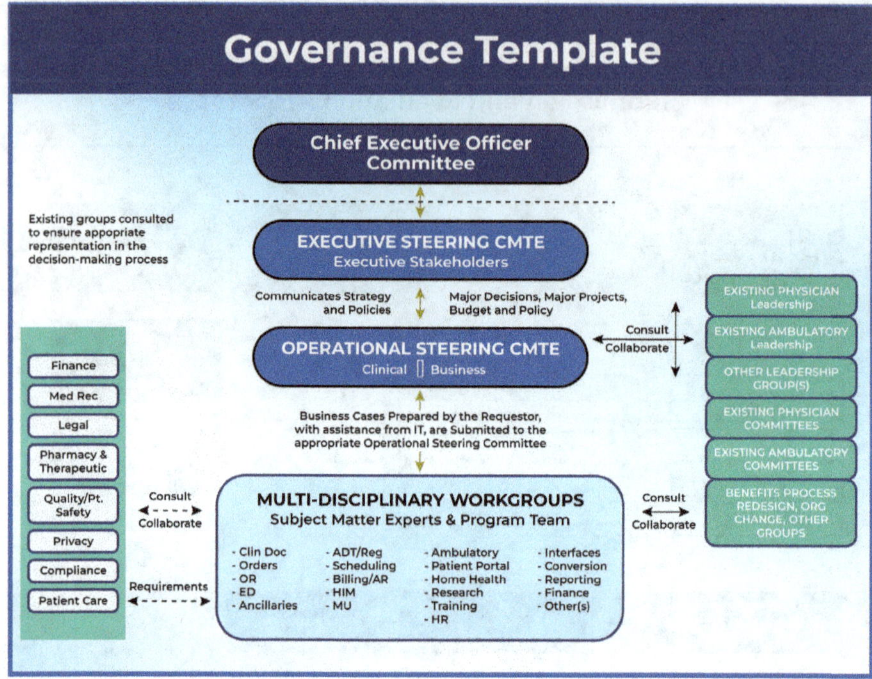

Security Oversight Group (SOG)
Meeting Frequency: Monthly; Ad-Hoc Meetings as Needed

Responsibilities	Participants
• Responsible for consistency of decisions across all business areas related to information security and privacy.	- Chief Information Officer
• Review security and privacy incidents for regulatory and information risk management.	- Chief Legal Officer & Privacy Officer - Chief Human Resources Officer - VP Internal Audit
• Review and discuss cybersecurity challanges and risk to the health system.	- VP Applications - Chief Information Security Officer
• Responsible for authorizing the development and implementation of information Security polices, standards, procedures and guidelines.	- Manager Internal Audit - Deputy Counsel Legal Officers - Others (Ad-Hoc as Needed)
• Review and approve proposed strategic initiatives to ensure they align with system enterprise strategies and methodologies.	

Figure 10.1. The 90 Day CIO Model ©

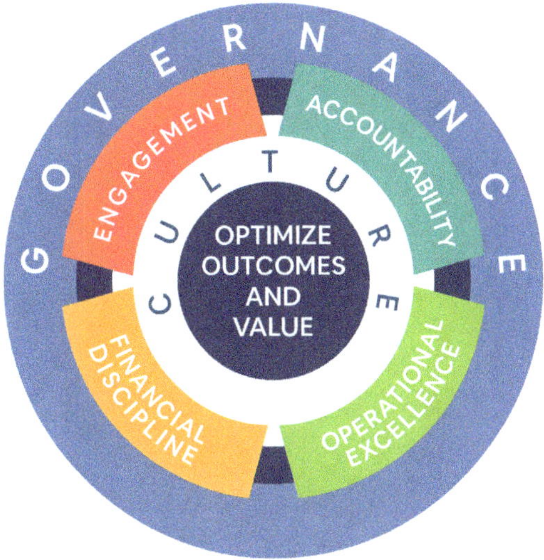
GOVERNANCE
CULTURE
ENGAGEMENT
ACCOUNTABILITY
FINANCIAL DISCIPLINE
OPERATIONAL EXCELLENCE
OPTIMIZE
OUTCOMES
AND
VALUE

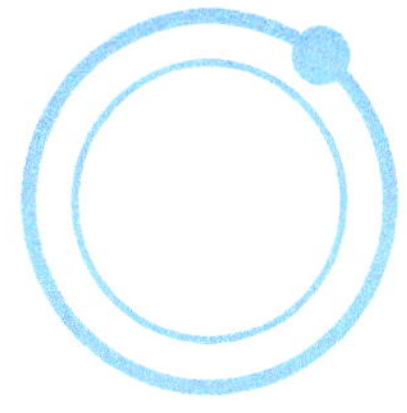

Appendix B:

All References

B, Cody. "10 Healthcare Technology Advancements in the Last Decade." ReferralMD, March 18, 2021. https://getreferralmd.com/2021/02/10-healthcare-technology-advancements-in-the-last-decade/.

"Best Technological Inventions in Last Decade That Changed Technology Sector: YTD." YourTechDiet, January 23, 2023. https://yourtechdiet.com/blogs/10-best-inventions-last-decade-technology/.

Capone, Anthony. "Council Post: The Future of Healthcare Technology." Forbes. Forbes Magazine, October 12, 2022. https://www.forbes.com/sites/forbestechcouncil/2022/01/11/the-future-of-healthcare-technology/?sh=2fcd3c3c4750.

Emmet O'Gara, EVP. "The Role of Population Health in Value-Based Care." Modern Healthcare, February 27, 2020. https://www.modernhealthcare.com/patient-care/role-population-health-value-based-care.

Erin McNemar, MPA. "What Is the Role of Data Analytics in Population Health Management?." HealthITAnalytics. HealthITAnalytics, February 1, 2023. https://healthitanalytics.com/features/whatistherole-ofdataanalytics-inpopulationhealthmanagement.

Evans, Christopher Riche. *The Making of the Micro: A History of the Computer*. New York: Van Nostrand Reinhold, 1981.

Farmanova, Elina, G. Ross Baker, and Deborah Cohen. "Combining Integration of Care and a Population Health Approach: A Scoping Review of Redesign Strategies and Interventions, and Their Impact." *International Journal of Integrated Care* 19, no. 2 (2019). https://doi.org/10.5334/ijic.4197.

Hewitt, Anne M., Julie L. Mascari, and Stephen L. Wagner. *Population Health Management: Strategies, Tools, Applications, and Outcomes*. New York, NY: Springer Publishing Company, LLC, 2022.

"IBM 5280." Wikipedia. Wikimedia Foundation, December 8, 2022. https://en.wikipedia.org/wiki/IBM_5280.

Kattan, Michael W., and Mark E. Cowen. *Encyclopedia of Medical Decision Making*. Thousand Oaks: SAGE Publications, Inc, 2009.

Nurse.com Powered by Relias. "Population Health Management Is about Teamwork." Nurse.com digital guides and publications. Nurse.com Powered by Relias, February 18, 2023. https://resources.nurse.com/training-days.

PatientEngagementHIT. "How Are Population Health, Patient Engagement Different?" PatientEngagementHIT, December 22, 2020. https://patientengagementhit.com/news/how-are-population-health-patient-engagement-different.

Reed, William J. "The Pareto, Zipf and Other Power Laws." *Economics Letters* 74, no. 1 (2001): 15–19. https://doi.org/10.1016/s0165-1765(01)00524-9.

"Social Determinants of Health." World Health Organization. World Health Organization. Accessed March 8, 2023. https://www.who.int/health-topics/social-determinants-of-health#tab=tab_1.

"What Is 'Perfect Information'?" Economy, February 24, 2017. https://www.ecnmy.org/learn/you/social-influences-culture-information/what-is-perfect-information/.

World Economic Forum. "These 10 Medical Breakthroughs Will Change the World." World Economic Forum, December 6, 2019. https://www.weforum.org/agenda/2019/12/10-ways-medical-innovation-will-transform-our-lives-over-the-next-decade/.

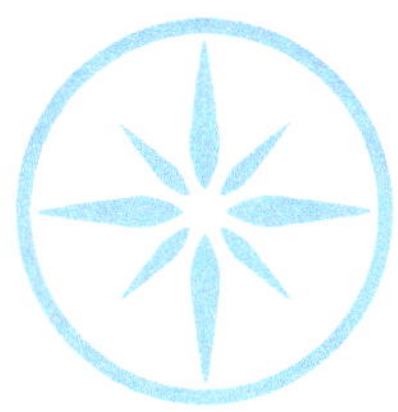

Acknowledgements

I am deeply grateful for the strong support I have received from numerous individuals throughout the process of writing this book. While it is impossible to acknowledge every single person, I would like to express my gratitude to a select few who have made significant contributions. Thank you to all who have supported me.

- ✦ **Bruce Johnson,** a dear friend since 1987 when he was the CIO of a hospital and my customer at IBM. He has held several CIO positions and is the founder and president of NJ Associates, a technology consulting firm based in New Jersey.

- ✦ **Dan Garrett,** a retired Partner and US Technology consulting Leader, and Healthcare Technology Consulting Leader at PwC. Dan helped me maintain a big-picture perspective throughout the writing process. He currently serves on the Board of Directors of multiple US companies.

- ✦ **Jessica Shure** and **Gerald (Butch) Hertkorn** from the Lehigh Valley Health Network, who shared their financial expertise.

- ✦ **Jim Rossiter**, an IBM colleague, and long-term friend who provided valuable feedback during the writing process. Jim has taught me the meaning of tenacity and perseverance with his entrepreneurial spirit.

- ✦ **Linda Gerber,** co-founder, and my partner at the Health Data Synthesis Institute (HDSI). She currently serves as the Chief Operating Officer and Technology Architect of HDSI and has been a trusted advisor for almost a decade.

- ✦ **Shri Ajvalia and the team at Keshri Publishing,** who were instrumental in transforming my thoughts and writings into the readable format that you see here.

- ✦ **Stephen O'Mahony**, MD, FACP, Senior Vice President and Chief Health Information Officer at RWJBarnabas Health. Stephen, a colleague, and friend of over a decade, provided invaluable clinical input and guidance.

To each of these individuals, I extend my heartfelt gratitude for their unwavering support, guidance, and contributions. Without them, this book would not have been possible.